Sugar Detox

FILIPPA SALOMONSSON

Sugar Detox

TRANSLATION: GUN PENHOAT

PHOTOGRAPHY: KARLA GARCIA AND ULRIKA POUSETTE

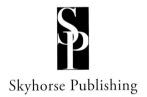

Skyhorse Publishing

Let go of your sugar dependency and create a healthy relationship with sugar!

Contents

CHAPTER 1: MY JOURNEY WITH SUGAR 7

CHAPTER 2: WHAT IS SUGAR? 17

Different sugars 19

How much sugar do you consume? 22

Food that controls us 26

CHAPTER 3: CLEAN EATING AND PERSONAL EATING HABITS 31

Clean eating 32

Personal eating habits 37

Three potential pitfalls 41

CHAPTER 4: YOUR SUGAR DETOX PROGRAM 45

Before you begin 48

Away from your kitchen 51

Mindful eating 57

Positive affirmations 58

Prep week 60

Week 1–Detox Week 62

Week 2– Nutrition Week 66

Week 3– Final Week 70

CHAPTER 5: RECIPES 75

Breakfast 78

Snacks 88

Lunch/Dinner 96

CHAPTER 6: LIVING A HEALTHY LIFESTYLE AFTER THE PROGRAM 125

First week after program's completion 128

Second week after program's completion 131

Healthy sweets 132

Healthy habits for life 140

Sources 142

Conversion Charts 143

THANK YOU! 144

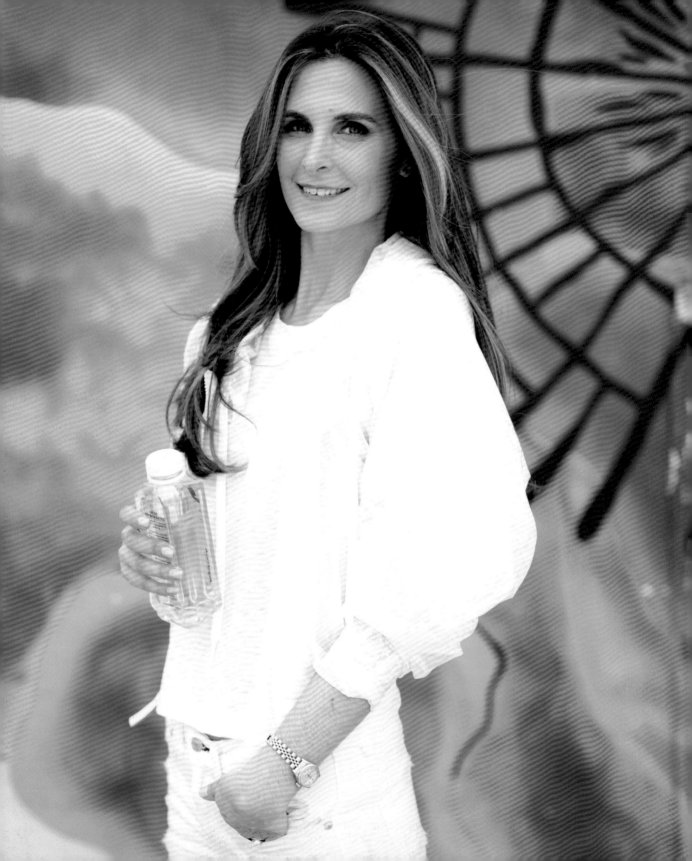

CHAPTER 1

MY Journey with Sugar

MY JOURNEY WITH SUGAR HAS NOT BEEN EASY. I ALWAYS THOUGHT I NEEDED A DAILY DOSE OF SUGAR TO FUNCTION. SUGAR WAS KIND OF LIKE A FLAKY FRIEND—ALWAYS THERE WHEN I NEEDED IT, BUT NEVER REALLY USEFUL. THIS IS MY PATH TOWARD ACHIEVING A HEALTHY RELATIONSHIP WITH SUGAR.

I'VE GONE THROUGH STRETCHES OF TIME WHEN I felt completely helpless in the face of sweets. I relied on sugar for a long time to satisfy my cravings, to cope with stress, and to feel joy and support. However, I never found what I was really looking for in sugar; instead, I uncovered it once sugar disappeared from my life. That's what it took for me to see the light! I realized I'd been using sugar as a tool for avoiding my emotions; it had become a handy crutch for not dealing with situations that required my attention and presence. Today, I'm free of sugar's stranglehold, and can enjoy treats without an anxiety-ridden debate raging in the back of my mind.

My journey with sugar has taken me far, and it's a wonderful feeling! I often wonder what made me put up with my dependency on it, but as I sit here writing this, I've come to understand why. I had to help myself so that I would be able to help others later on. Today I'm a holistic health coach for women of all ages. The word "holistic" highlights the fact that my take on health comes from a broad perspective. I want to understand and take into consideration all aspects of daily living and their effects on us.

In spite of my earlier reliance on sugar, I've always had a keen interest in whole foods and health; I became a vegetarian at age fifteen. A few years ago, once I'd decided to adopt a completely healthy lifestyle, it wasn't hard to sell my PR firm in Manhattan and come back to Sweden, my accrued knowledge and experience in tow. Long before my return to Stockholm, I had decided that my life's work was in finding a way back to natural nutrition, both for myself and for others.

But this has not been an easy task, since sugar was my drug of choice. My addiction to the sweet white substance was both conscious and subconscious, and I needed my daily dose to function. I turned to sugar for lots of reasons, and sugar was always at hand.

Sugar was my sneaky accomplice—always good to me, but never good *for* me. It offered me temporary solace, but I always felt let down afterward. Nevertheless, I held on to my sugar pal for almost eighteen years. Looking back, I sometimes wonder how my body has been affected all the sugar I ingested over what amounts to a total of 6,570 days. I might not have indulged in sweets every single day, but it was close enough, and certainly in sufficient quantities to create an addiction to them.

Some of my childhood memories consist of my brothers and I getting off the school bus, running toward our front door, ditching our backpacks in the hallway, and rushing into the kitchen to look for treats. My mother never let us have a lot of unhealthy food, so we had to uncover her hiding spots when she wasn't looking. Afterward, I would immediately head to my room to scarf down what I had managed to sneak away in my pocket. This is where my unhealthy relationship with sugar began to take root. I always thought I had things under control, when in fact it was sugar that had me under its spell.

A candy-filled childhood

When I was seven, my parents decided to move the family from Kungsbacka, on the west coast of Sweden, to New York. My Swedish teacher had warned me about the city before we crossed the Atlantic. According to her, everything was much larger in the US, and there was so much more of everything. She was indeed correct. There was no comparison to what you could get in Kungsbacka. As if that weren't enough, access to everything was much easier, too—there seemed to be twice the choice, and all the stores were open at least one hour past my regular bedtime.

It didn't take long for me to realize that the contents of my school friends' lunch boxes were different from mine. They had treats such as Fruit Roll-Ups, cookies, sodas, and chips. My cheese sandwiches and sliced apples were boring, and embarrassed me in front of my new friends, so unbeknownst to my mother, I began to trade her carefully wrapped lunches for my school's processed sugar bombs. After all, these options were cheap—everything cost less than a dollar—an easy amount of money to come by for a seven-year-old, as there were always a couple of quarters rolling around in the bottom of

I NEEDED MY DAILY DOSE TO FUNCTION — AT TIMES IN LARGER AMOUNTS, SOMETIMES LESSER.

my backpack. My friends weren't aware of the Swedish concept of "Saturday sweets," and naturally I found "every day sweets" a far more attractive concept than our family's once-a-week pick n' mix. Furthermore, in those days our traditional Saturday sweets were, for instance, two round salty "S" coins, a Snuff lollipop filled with licorice powder, and a licorice rope, all contained within a bag no bigger than the size of my palm.

As I mentioned earlier, there was just so much more of everything in the States, including television programs. I went from watching the Swedish show *Bolibompa* a few times a week to constantly surfing between the twenty-five American channels aimed at kids. Between animated cartoons, Kellogg's held me rapt with their ads for Frosted Flakes, Pop-Tarts, and Eggos. Swedish laws restrict multinational corporations from influencing children with direct advertising, but in the States an "anything goes" mantra reigns, so children tend to be swayed from a very early age.

I was oblivious to my addiction to sugar, but I remember constantly searching for something sweet to eat. It wasn't merely a physiological need that I sought to placate, but an emotional one, as well. I grew up with three siblings, and while we were deeply loved by our parents, we weren't always given the time and encouragement we needed. I often found comfort in food rather than from my parents. I used food to suppress what I didn't want, or lacked the fortitude, to deal with. This was the start of a long and complicated journey.

My first diet

I hated my body as a teenager, so my next food phase—dieting—began around the time I was seventeen. I couldn't understand why my thighs wouldn't fit into my best friend's cool skinny jeans, or why my belly wasn't as flat as Heidi Klum's when she modeled bikinis. Instead, I was destined to have curves, which didn't match up with my idea of the "perfect body."

I was disappointed and dissatisfied, so one sleepless night I decided to do something about it. I was alone in Paris for a few weeks for work, which meant I had complete control over my food intake. And the best plan that I could find to lose weight? SlimFast—that was my very first diet. I traded all my meals for 200 calories' worth of "chocolate cookie dough bars" and strawberry shakes. I felt incredibly pleased when I flew back to Sweden a few weeks later and my grandmother worriedly asked me why

SUGAR WAS KIND OF LIKE A FLAKY
FRIEND—ALWAYS THERE WHEN I NEEDED, IT
BUT NEVER REALLY USEFUL.

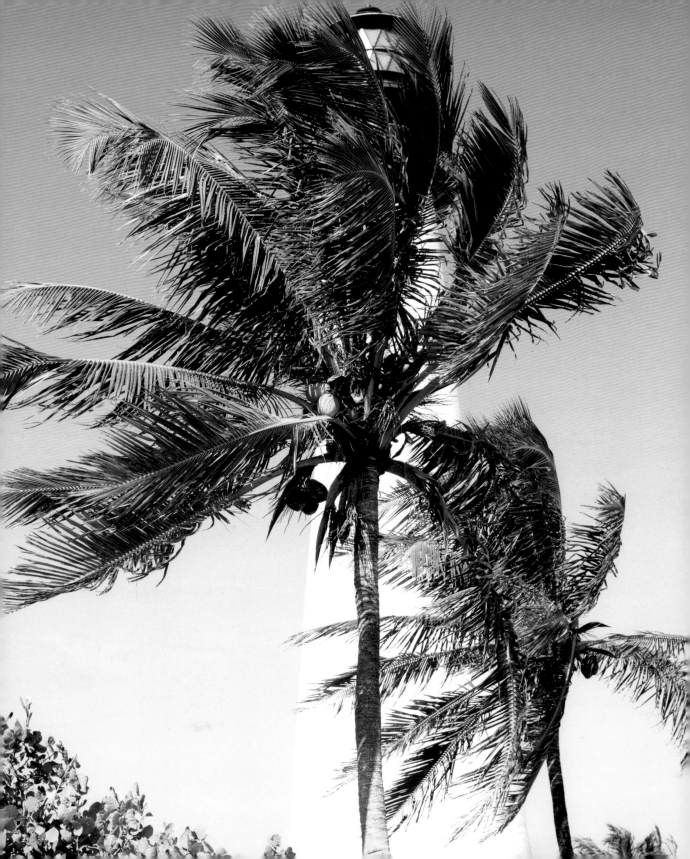

I was so thin. *Mission accomplished*, I thought. It didn't matter at all that my skin was gray, that I had dark circles under my eyes, that my temper was on a roller coaster, and that there was no way I could exercise (my head would spin). But, hey—the jeans fit!

It would take me another ten years to realize that a real approach to health wasn't compatible with calorie counting, but with learning how to create a new relationship with my body, my feelings, with food in general, and, yes—with sugar.

An active lifestyle, but with an unhappy stomach

My time at the University of Miami meant, among other things, Frappuccinos at Starbucks, sugar bomb smoothies at Jamba Juice, and "apple-tinis" at the Shore Club—all containing hidden sugars that I paid no heed to. It's a good thing drinks on South Beach didn't come with nutrition labels. I did have a vague idea of the sugar content in everything I ate, but my main focus during those years was on counting calories. Don't ask me my rationale—I really have no idea. I tried hard to keep my eyes open during lectures, but sudden drops in energy pulled me down. The constant roller-coaster ride of my blood-sugar levels made it challenging to concentrate on tasks at hand. At times I would pretend to rub my eyes, which was just an excuse to close my eyes for a few minutes without the teacher taking notice. Thankfully, my natural perfectionism saved me during those years at college—I needed to be the best and most accomplished. Nothing else was acceptable.

My body resisted, but I refused to look deeper into my problems; I simply shut my eyes and tried other quick fixes in an attempt to solve symptoms. My biggest issue? Irritable bowel syndrome, more commonly referred to as IBS. My guts were inflamed from all the sugar and processed food they had to deal with; they were no doubt wondering where all the fiber, micronutrients, and chlorophyll had vanished. My belly staged a mutiny and manifested its displeasure by causing me a lot of pain at least six to eight times a year. My doctors blamed my ills on stress, and recommended that I slow down, but no one really took the time to uncover the real reason behind my complaints; perhaps it was easier to mask the symptoms with fiber tablets.

It was up to me to take a closer look at things, so I made my body my guinea pig. Should I stop drinking milk or stop eating white bread? Perhaps I shouldn't eat so late at night or perhaps my portions are too big? I finally got to know and understand my body via process of elimination. I was finally able to pinpoint where my issues had begun—sugar, which had created all these problems and brought about this very painful period in my life. Peace and quiet were all well and good, but my insides were irritated the most by the white sugar that casually passed through my stomach uninvited. A short visit from sugar could cause an inflammation that lasted for days. Now I had my answer, but my desire to resist sugar was not as strong as I wished it could be. Even with all this newfound knowledge, I still couldn't let go of sugar altogether. Well, that's not true—I couldn't let go of it at all.

A hectic work schedule

After graduating from the University of Miami, I boarded the first flight to New York for a job interview at one of the world's largest PR firms. I was picked out from a field of two hundred candidates, but minutes before signing the contract I realized that my heart wasn't in it, and that it wasn't the right choice for me. A short time later, I joined a small event-planning company. My first project was opening the Playboy Club at the Palms Hotel in Las Vegas. At twenty-one years old, I stepped right into a world of phones ringing nonstop, late nights at the office with a bag of peanut M&M's on my desk, and being under constant pressure to seal the deal. But no matter how hard I tried, I could not be Miss Perfect.

Constantly stressed out, I went back to sugar for pleasure, relaxation, and a break from the pulse of the big city. I often didn't get home until 10.00 p.m., where I searched the kitchen high and low for chocolate-covered raisins, "natural" brownies from Whole Foods, or raspberry sorbet from Häagen-Dazs. Ashamed of my eating habits, I typically ate alone and only when my roommate couldn't see me. Mentally exhausted after a day in the world of public relations, sugar was my way of handling the daily stresses and pressures of my job.

My body began to feel very uncomfortable from the extra twenty-five pounds that had packed themselves upon my person. I didn't look good anymore. I didn't enjoy life at its fullest. Sugar prevented me from taking advantage of everything that the Big Apple had to offer. My sample of its myriad opportunities was far too small due to my relationship with food. I finally hit my lowest point, and realized that I couldn't continue like this any longer. I had to let go and start fresh.

Toward a healthier life

During this time, the self-help book *The Secret* was a hot topic of conversation over Sunday brunches. It's about the laws of attraction, as in, everything you say and think will come back to you in one way or another. One day, I decided to read the book and apply its philosophy—even though my inner skeptic tried hard to make itself heard. I created a large mood board; the book recommends using this as a tool to make your dream life manifest itself more quickly. To create a motivating collage, I cut out and pinned up pictures of healthy-looking meals and girls from magazines, and hung it on the wall over my bed. Of all the images that inspired me on this new board, I remember the phrase "healthy for life," written out in a large turquoise font, most vividly. This has been my motto ever since! Let me also point out that I have been granted everything else I asked from life after that day—even the love of my life.

Let's keep going until we find ourselves in Stockholm, about seven years later. I left my unhealthy relationship with sugar behind when I moved to Sweden. Today, I have a different attitude toward sweets. I don't allow sugar to take control of me as it did before. I listen to my body's signals, and know how to respond if my consumption of sugar begins to increase. I now have a normal relationship with sugar, which is not as difficult to establish as you might think.

This was a glimpse into my journey with sugar—we'll cover the rest of the stretch together. I will guide you step-by-step over the next few weeks until you reach a new understanding of sugar. So, are you ready to empty the pantry of all candy and treats? Good! Throw all of it out immediately, and let's begin your first official day of sugar detox. Welcome to change—for good.

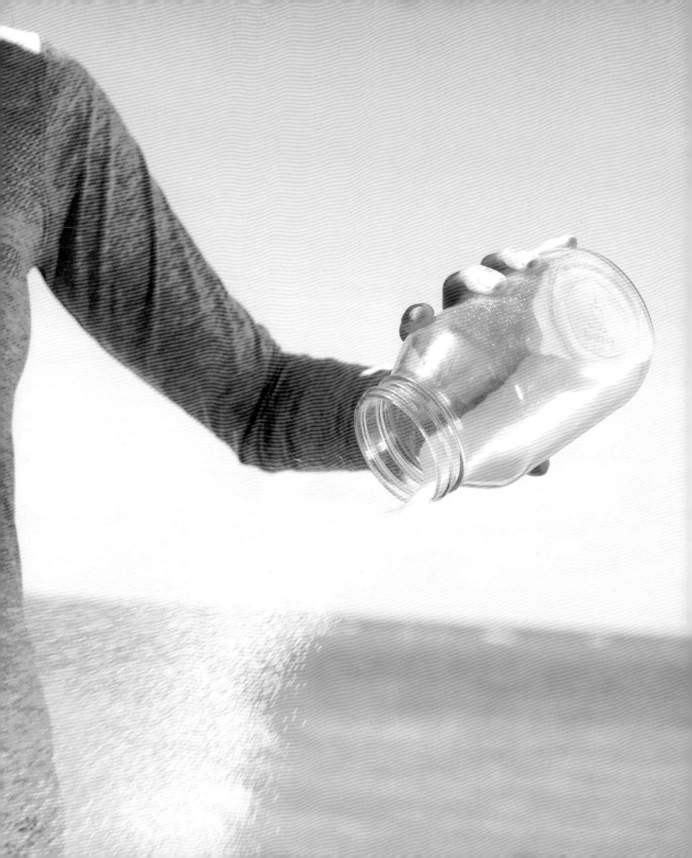

CHAPTER 2

What is Sugar?

TEST YOUR SENSITIVITY TO SUGAR. GET TO KNOW MORE ABOUT SUGAR, WHY IT IS UNHEALTHY, AND WHY A SUGAR DETOX IS SO GOOD FOR YOU. HERE YOU CAN CALCULATE HOW MUCH SUGAR YOU CONSUME EACH DAY. THESE FACTS AREN'T ALL SWEET!

DO YOU FEEL YOUR ENERGY FLAGGING IN THE AFTERNOON? Do you crave a sweet treat after lunch? Do you find it hard to enjoy a single piece of chocolate but easy to keep eating them until the dish is completely empty? If you answered yes to these questions, it is more than likely that you have a sensitivity to sugar. There's nothing wrong with that that, considering how much sugar we consume on a daily basis—both consciously and unconsciously. We yearn for something sweet not only because it tastes good, but because it signals pleasure by releasing dopamine, a natural "feel-good" hormone. But the dopamine signals decline when we eat too much sugar, causing us to crave ever-larger quantities of sweets to create the same effect. In this case, a strong will is not enough to get rid of sugar addiction because our biochemical processes are in charge! Sugar behaves like any other chemical substance when ingested; in the end it works like a drug. Did you know that it is eight times harder to give up sugar than it is to quit cocaine?

You're certainly aware of the many negative ways sugar affects you and your body. Whose dentist hasn't told us that we must reduce the amount of candy we eat? Who hasn't connected sugar to added inches on waist, thighs, and backside? However, do you know what sugar really is, and how it behaves in your body? Perhaps not completely? Let's take a closer look. First, take the following quiz to check your status.

Quiz: Are you sensitive to sugar?

Take this test to see if you exhibit sensitivity to sugar. Answer "yes" or "no" to the following questions.

1. Do you crave sugar after every meal?
2. Are you tired in the afternoon, and often feel the need to eat something sweet as a pick-me-up?
3. Do you feel that you can't always control your craving for sweets?
4. At night, do you raid the pantry in search of chocolate or other types of candy?
5. Are you constantly (or at least several times a day) preoccupied by thoughts of when and how you can eat something sweet?

6. Do you find it difficult to resist buying candy when you're shopping for groceries?
7. Do you have trouble resisting cakes and cookies at your workplace?
8. Do you reward yourself with sweets?
9. Do you get irritated when you eat or drink something sweet? Or do you get bad-tempered when you don't eat something sweet?
10. Do you eat sweets even if you're not hungry?
11. Do you use sweets for comfort when you feel lonely, bored, sad, or unloved?
12. Do you sometimes hide to eat sweets?
13. Do you feel bloated after eating too much sugar?
14. Is it difficult for you to say no to sweets when they're offered?
15. Do you have difficulty stopping once you've started eating sweets?
16. Do you occasionally feel anxious after drinking a soda or eating candy?
17. Do you cope with stress by eating sweets?
18. Do you feel envious of people who can control their intake of sweets?

If you answered yes to three or more questions, it's more than likely that you suffer from sensitivity to sugar. But, fear not: in three weeks' time you'll be able to look back on this quiz, and hopefully feel free of sugar's control over you.

DIFFERENT SUGARS

There are five main types of sugar. Our focus is on fructose, as it is the big baddie here.

Fructose—Found in (among other things) fruit, candy, white sugar, and soda.

Glucose—Found in (among other things) fruit, berries, white sugar, and vegetables.

Lactose—Found in dairy products in varying amounts. For lactose to break down and be digested, the enzyme lactase must be present in the intestine.

Sucrose—A carbohydrate consisting of one glucose molecule and one fructose molecule. Sucrose is the name of regular white sugar.

Maltose—A carbohydrate present in malted drinks and beer.

27 reasons
to decrease your sugar intake

We've all heard that sugar is bad for you, but what are its negative effects? Sugar can:

1. Compromise the immune system
2. Create inflammation
3. Contribute to weight gain
4. Increase the risk of cellulite
5. Cause and aid the growth of cancer
6. Contribute to premature aging and wrinkles
7. Cause dental cavities
8. Compromise your body's pH level
9. Cause cardiovascular disease
10. Affect insulin levels, which can eventually lead to diabetes
11. Create unbalanced intestinal flora, leading to inflammation-causing bacteria and constipation
12. Disturb the balance of minerals and their beneficial interactions, which can interfere with the body's absorption of minerals and cause mineral insufficiency
13. Cause anxiety, difficulty in concentrating, irritation, depression, and fatigue
14. Impair vision
15. Contribute to autoimmune diseases such as arthritis, asthma, and multiple sclerosis
16. Lower vitamin E levels
17. Impede the absorption of proteins
18. Weaken DNA structure
19. Cause headaches and migraines
20. Cause dermatological upsets, such as acne
21. Increase the risk for irritable bowel syndrome (IBS), and irritate the digestive system
22. Impair liver function as much as alcohol
23. Create a substance dependency
24. Affect sleep quality
25. Impair sexual desire
26. Speed up the rate of aging
27. Increase risk of infertility

Glucose, yes please—fructose, no thanks!

Not all sugar is bad. Our bodies need certain sugars, but not just any type. For instance, we need glucose. Glucose is the primary source of energy for all our bodily functions. It is the main source of energy for the brain. Every living cell contains glucose. The body typically processes glucose first, and if we don't get enough of it from our food, our body will make it. Glucose can be found in fruits, vegetables, and quinoa.

Fructose, on the other hand, is something our bodies don't need to function. The body works perfectly well—even better, actually—without it. Only the liver is able to break down fructose, and only in limited quantities. The liver can cope with a certain amount, and any excess is converted to glycogen, which is stored until needed. When the liver is saturated with glycogen and there is no more room for incoming fructose, the fructose is then converted to fat. So don't shy away from fat; fat is not your enemy—fructose is. Fructose is in white sugar or added to different beverages. Too much fructose doesn't just make your pants tight at the waist; it also affects your health in many other ways. Go ahead and check out the list on the opposite page, where you'll find twenty-seven reasons why you should curtail your intake of sugar.

Let's recap! As pointed out earlier, we use glucose for quick energy, while fructose is converted to fatty acids, which the body stores as fat. Now, this doesn't mean that the body needs a large amount of glucose, either—everything in moderation. You don't have to be Einstein to understand which changes need to take place. But don't panic, we are on this journey together, taking it one step at a time. The most important thing is to decrease the amount of sugar we eat by avoiding sweet baked goods, sweetened beverages, and candy.

Do you sometimes have trouble recognizing your body's natural hunger signals? This is a common side effect of ingesting too much sugar. Well-known pediatric endocrinologist and sugar specialist Dr. Robert Lustig explains: "Glucose suppresses the hunger hormone ghrelin and stimulates leptin, which suppresses your appetite. Fructose has no effect on ghrelin and interferes with your brain's communication with leptin."

As a consequence, the body doesn't signal when it has reached satiety. You can continue to eat more and more without noticing any red lights or blinking stop signals from your body. That's why it's so easy to go through an entire bowl of candy while watching your favorite episode of *Sex and the City*. But the body reacts differently when we eat glucose, and it emits clear signals to stop eating once it has had enough.

SUGAR AND OUR HORMONES

Sugar affects our hormones, which can affect our sensitivity to insulin, a hormone that works as a key to open our cells so they can take in glucose from the blood. This glucose is then used as energy. When we consume an excess of sugary treats, our insulin sensitivity decreases (which is bad). The body then requires greater amounts of insulin in order to open the cells to take in energy. Too much insulin can cause blood glucose levels to drop and bring on insulin resistance. Low blood glucose levels bring on sugar cravings, which often happen after eating sugar-rich foods.

Insulin is critical for the body, so eating lots of sugar for prolonged periods of time can compromise our sensitivity to it. This can result in diabetes and other negative health outcomes. Please keep this in mind!

Studies show when cortisol or stress hormone levels are too elevated, we are highly likely to eat more food, especially in the form of comfort foods, as Dr. Robert Lustig calls them. This means we consume far more calories than what we need; it's entirely natural to seek out a trusty chocolate bar when we're stressed or fatigued. You see, even too little sleep can elevate cortisol levels, so the hunger hormone, ghrelin, increases while the satiety hormone, leptin (which tells you that you are full), decreases and insulin resistance is impaired. Studies have shown that missing as little as two hours sleep out of the recommended eight hours can have undesirable consequences. So make sure you get enough shut-eye to keep cravings at bay!

HOW MUCH SUGAR DO YOU CONSUME?

According to a Swedish nutrition study, women and men consume approximately eighty-eight pounds, the equivalent of ten thousand teaspoons of sugar, per year. I'm not surprised. For example, if you drink 33 cl (11 oz) of soda, you're consuming ten teaspoons of sugar. Do you sprinkle a small packet of raisins over your breakfast muesli? That's eight teaspoons of sugar right there. It bears repeating: we can cope with a certain amount sugar, but we have to become conscious of how much of it we actually consume.

Naturally, you're wondering how much sugar per day is considered too much. According to the World Health Organization, "Only 5 percent of the daily energy intake should consist of added or 'free' sugars. That is the equivalent of five to six teaspoons (25 grams, or 0.88 ounces) for women and seven to eight teaspoons (35 grams, or 1.23 ounces) for men." I recommend a daily "added" sugar intake of no more than 6 teaspoons (approximately 25 grams, or 0.88 ounces). Sugar isn't detrimental in small doses, but it is in larger amounts. Do you have an idea how much sugar you eat per day, week, month, or year? Even if you are somewhat conscious of which foods contain added sugar, perhaps you're a bit hazy on the exact quantity. Aside from being in candy, sodas, and pastries, sugar also hides in a long list of other foods. Did you know that ketchup and bouillon cubes contain sugar? That it pops up in yogurt and balsamic vinegar, too? You really don't need to eat many regular ingredients before your body has reached the recommended amount. Perhaps your lunch had enough sugar in it to cover the entire day!

Now it's time to roll up your sleeves and start calculating how much sugar you are ingesting. Are you ready to calculate how many teaspoons of sugar are actually passing across your lips? Okay then, let's get to it! You'll see below how to convert grams to teaspoons; on the next page you'll find a four-step quiz and a guide listing the sugar content in some regular, everyday foods.

CONVERTING GRAMS TO TEASPOONS
One teaspoon of sugar is the equivalent of sixteen calories.

1 gram of sugar = approx. ¼ teaspoon
4 grams of sugar = approx. 1 teaspoon
8 grams of sugar = approx. 2 teaspoons
12 grams of sugar = approx. 3 teaspoons
16 grams of sugar = approx. 4 teaspoons
20 grams of sugar = approx. 5 teaspoons

QUIZ: HOW MUCH SUGAR DO YOU EAT ON A DAILY BASIS?

Step 1: Keep a food diary for one day
Don't cheat! All meals must be included, even snacks and beverages. If you prefer, you can write down several days' worth of meals to get a more accurate end figure. This step is an honest evaluation of your food habits without being judgmental. You'll simply increase your awareness, which in turn will enable you to make better choices from here on out.

Step 2: Write down every gram of sugar in all your meals
Concentrate on candies, fruit, dried fruit, processed foods, and dairy products. Don't forget to double-check for hidden sugars. You don't have to spend as much time on natural ingredients such as fish, quinoa, vegetables etc. Consult your foods' nutrition facts to calculate your intake of sugar. Use the next page's table to calculate for fresh food, such as fruit and vegetables.

Step 3: Convert grams to teaspoons
It's easier to visualize quantities of sugar by using teaspoons instead of grams. Use the preceding page's table to calculate and write down how many teaspoons of sugar you eat and drink daily.

Step 4: Add it all up!
Multiply your final total by seven to see how much sugar you consume in a week; multiply it by thirty to get the amount for the month. Finally, multiply it by 365 to get an idea of the quantity over a period of a year. Don't forget that we often eat a wide variety of foods, so the tally is an approximate number. Regardless, is the amount you ended up with more or less than you expected? The recommendation is six teaspoons of added sugar a day. How do you compare?

What is the fructose content of sweet-tasting food? How much sugar is it, when converted to teaspoons?

RAW PRODUCT (100g/3.5 oz)	FRUCTOSE %	TOTAL SUGAR	SUGAR IN TSP
Agave syrup	85	72	18
Orange	2.7	8.9	2.2
Banana	2.7	13.5	3.4
Blueberries	2.9	6.4	1.6
Croissant	<0.1	0.3	0.1
Raspberries	2.2	4.1	1.0
Honey	41.4	80.8	20.2
Ketchup	3.8	19.2	4.8
Kiwi fruit	3.4	6.8	1.7
Soda (Coca-Cola)	3.4	10.9	2.7
Carrots	1.4	5.4	1.4
Raisins	28.9	60.1	15.0
Spinach	0.1	0.3	0.1
Watermelon	2.3	7.1	1.8
White, processed sugar	50	99.9	25.0
Sweet white wine	3.3	6.0	1.6
Apple	3.5	6.6	1.7

FOOD THAT CONTROLS US

Candy

It's difficult to classify candy, as there are so many varieties, each with different ingredients. But most pieces in your bag have one common denominator—sugar! Not in small quantities, either.

Sweden's love affair with candy began in the seventeenth century. Nordic countries were ruled by kings and the aristocracy, but the power of candy suppliers still lay in the distant future. Swedes were first introduced to drinking chocolate in the 1600s; today they're the world's most voracious consumers of candy, leading other countries with a whopping 17 kg (37.5 lbs) per person—each year! That's twice the average of the European Union.

But what is it that Swedish people are gorging on? How many of them do you believe actually check the list of ingredients on a bag of jelly beans on a Saturday night? There isn't room here to list and analyze the ingredients in all your personal favorite treats, but one thing is for sure—they are all sugar bombs. Candy can also contain gelatin (pig parts and other slaughter by-products), which take on many different forms to create the right consistency. If you don't eat meat, you might need to be vigilant. Check the list of ingredients carefully next time you enjoy a sweet treat.

Soda

The amount of sugar in a soda is absolutely stunning. An ordinary can of Coca-Cola contains 35 grams (1.25 oz) of sugar, which equals approximately nine teaspoons. A 1½ liter (1.5 quart) bottle of Fanta has 167 grams (5.89 oz) of sugar, which comes to almost forty-two teaspoons. We're way over the recommended daily allowance of six teaspoons. There is nothing refreshing about those facts. You can do yourself and your family a huge favor by reducing your soda intake.

Cookies and pastries

Sometimes it's difficult to estimate the sugar content of baked goods and cookies. This is especially true if they're bought in a bakery, and the cakes are bundled into a nice bag that lacks any nutritional information. When we're offered a pastry, we hardly ever ask how much sugar the item contains.

Instead, we politely drink our cup of coffee and eat the bun without question. Things are easier when you undergo a sugar detox because there's no need to ask for the sugar content in products.

But to prepare for the future, it's a good idea to become more conscious of what you eat, and realize that you really don't have to accept pastries or cookies merely out of politeness. You can simply accept the proffered cup of coffee.

My tip? Bake at home! There are lots of great options for which you'll know exactly what you're eating and what you're offering. You'll find my favorite sweets on pages 132 to 139. They're loaded with nutrients and delicious flavor, all without any white sugar.

OUT WITH SUGAR AND IN WITH NUTRITION

It can be a bit nerve-racking to cut out one specific ingredient or food group from one's diet. It can cause unpleasant and intrusive thoughts, but there's no other option if we want to get rid of our sugar sensitivity. It is necessary to eliminate all sugar during this period. When you've abused something you need a period of total abstinence to reset and start anew. As with an alcoholic who cannot drink just one drink, as this will put him or her right back in the grips of dependency, you'll have to cut sugar out completely for a while to rid yourself of your addiction. It'll be much easier to handle after three weeks, and you may not even want to eat sugar once you've experienced how good your body feels without it—it's the best feeling in the world! You'll be able to decline the coffee break treats at work. You'll walk home from the grocery store, bags full of healthy, nourishing foods after having ignored those candy bars that got routinely slipped into your shopping cart almost every time before your detox program. You'll feel so proud. You'll feel such power and so much respect for your body. Sugar owns this power at the moment, so take it back.

Pay attention to everything that is positive during this journey: all the wholesome, delicious recipes you're going to try out; your feeling of freedom from sugar addiction; your newfound knowledge that will strengthen you along the way; and all the assistance you are offering to your body so it can do its work. Think of all the good things you're adding to your life, and not about all the things you're feeling deprived of. Perhaps you might even forget about sugar altogether once you focus on the menu's colorful dishes. You will also enjoy healthy carbohydrates, fats, and protein to quell any sugar cravings and make your sugar detox as easy as possible.

NUTRIENTS AND SUGAR

CARBOHYDRATES

Don't be afraid of carbohydrates—they're fuel that provides energy for your body. You just have to eat the right kind, so concentrate on vegetables, nuts, lentils, beans, millet, sweet potatoes, buckwheat, barley, and oats. Popcorn also happens to be a great carbohydrate option, and is nice to have on hand for cozy evenings.

FATS

You will not get fat from fat. As we discussed earlier, it's sugar that is fattening. (Nevertheless, you can't eat fat in great amounts—everything within reason, as with anything else.) In fact, fat will make you feel satiated and satisfied. You can calm sugar cravings by eating healthy fats that are found in avocado, chia seeds, salmon, nuts, olive oil, and coconut oil. The body needs fat for energy, healthy skin, and optimal function of cells, nerves, brain, and heart, among other things.

PROTEIN

Protein also helps to curb sugar cravings. Try to include some protein with each meal to keep your blood sugars in balance, and for satiety. Excellent vegetarian sources of protein include eggs from free-range chickens, quinoa, nuts, beans, cheese, yogurt, hemp seed, pumpkin seeds, and sunflower seeds. There is also protein in fish, poultry, and meat. A good tip is to eat protein at breakfast, and again as part of an afternoon snack, for an even keel.

SUGAR: A SUMMARY

Remember the most important thing here is to reduce your intake of fructose, as it overloads the liver and can lead you to pack on the pounds. This means you must avoid refined white sugar, soda, candy, and sweetened baked goods.

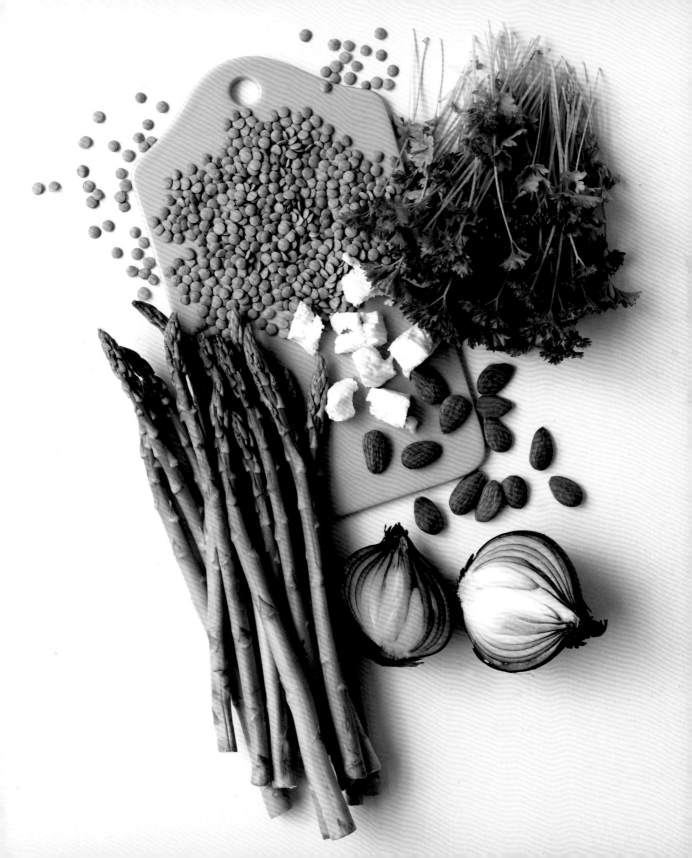

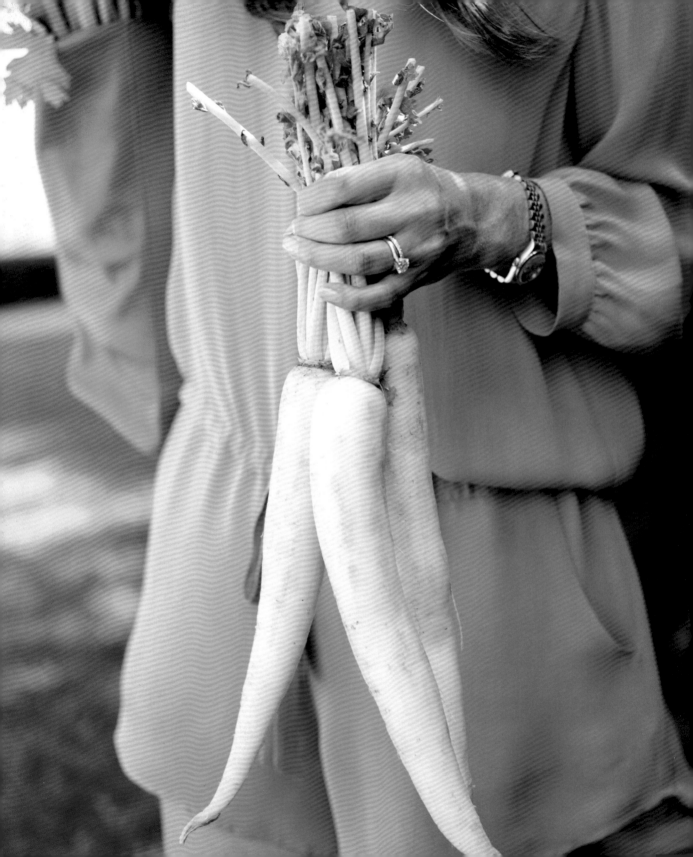

CHAPTER 3

Clean Eating and Personal Eating Habits

FOOD IS A PERSONAL MATTER, BUT EVERYONE WOULD FEEL MUCH BETTER IF THEY FOLLOWED A FEW BASIC RULES: EAT UNPROCESSED, CLEAN, SEASONAL, ORGANIC, AND GREEN FOODS AS OFTEN POSSIBLE. HERE YOU'LL LEARN WHAT IT MEANS TO EAT CLEAN, AND HOW YOU CAN ADJUST YOUR NUTRITION TO SUIT YOUR BODY'S NEEDS.

I DON'T BELIEVE IN DIETING. I'm also not a fan of quick weight loss solutions. If we take care to eat a variety of clean, unprocessed, and nutritionally balanced food, everything falls into place of its own accord. The body knows how much it's supposed to weigh, but it needs the right tools to reach that optimal number—tools in the form of food. However, weight is not the most important thing, or even something that I zero in on when I coach my clients. For many, the scale has become a starring role in their lives, to the detriment of other aspects of themselves that are far more important.

Sometimes food and weight take up so much of our attention that it prevents us from living our lives to the fullest. Many people avoid situations, meetings, and experiences because they suffer from low energy; they're on strict dietary programs; they battle constant sugar cravings; they exercise "bad food discipline"; and put forth a thousand other excuses that are directly tied to food. It's extremely exhausting and boring, isn't it? Sugar throws a big shadow, but in this section we're going to deal with the foods you can eat—not the foods to avoid.

CLEAN EATING

What does it mean to eat clean? To answer this question, I have divided it into several categories. It's all about thinking simply and using fundamental principles that humans have been following through the ages, before we started to process and destroy our foods' main ingredients.

We are supposed to eat food that is life sustaining and fresh, not sprayed with toxins—food that won't keep for months but will spoil naturally. Did you hear about Swedish raw-foods luminary Karin Haglund's hamburger experiment? She kept a McDonald's hamburger meal for six years, and it looked exactly as if it had been made today. Yuck. We have to wake up and become cognizant of what we chew, swallow, and use to build new cells, so let's back up and start our journey from the very beginning. Does that sound good to you? Let's do it.

KEEP IT WHOLE

The food you eat should remain as close to how nature intended it to be. It should, if at all possible, be eaten in the state it was found.

For example, there is a difference between a newly harvested green soybean and packaged processed soy milk, and the body reacts differently to the two. One becomes a friend that helps to build the body; the other turns into an enemy that the body doesn't recognize. The body is miraculous—it's constantly at work. If it feels threatened by a certain food, it can call for backup—i.e., the immune system. However, the immune system has more important jobs to do than clean out your morning Vanilla Light Frappuccino Blended Coffee. It had hoped for a green smoothie around 8 a.m. so it could continue to neutralize the beginnings of that cold you picked up while you were riding the bus.

Become aware of where your food is coming from and which manufacturing processes it has been subjected to. Eat food that has taken the shortest route to your plate.

UNPROCESSED

Processed food is food that has been industrially manufactured. It is food that is not in its original state and often contains more than two ingredients. If you turn over a bag of frozen blueberries and compare its nutritional information with that of a frozen dinner, you'll see that the blueberries contain only one ingredient while the processed, single serving meal can contain up to fifty separate ingredients. Even I, as a health coach, sometimes have trouble deciphering all the complicated terms on the packaging, and that is something the food industry is fully aware of. It's not enough that you have to be your own physician, but you also have to don Sherlock Holmes's deerstalker while grocery shopping. Processed grocery items often contain chemically created ingredients such as artificial coloring, artificial flavors, unhealthy vegetable oils, trans-fatty acids, and preservatives. These can have harmful and damaging effects on the body, either immediately or at some point in the future. Did you know that 74 percent of all prepackaged foods contain added sugar?

It's easier to head straight to the fruit and vegetable aisles! You don't have to worry that the organically grown beets will cause disease. Eating raw food became very trendy a few years ago, but you don't have to follow a 100-percent raw food diet to reap its benefits. I recommend that one third of your food be not heated above 104°F (40°C). When food is cooked, many important and heat-sensitive nutrients could be destroyed, and thus change the chemical makeup of ingredients. These are life-sustaining nutrients that your body needs. When you consume highly processed food you might miss out on a lot of nutrients, which in turn can lead to overeating. This might be a reaction to not getting enough nutrients, if you constantly feel hungry. Freshly squeezed and cold pressed juices, as well as smoothies, are a great way to meet that one-third raw food quota per day.

THE 80/20 RULE

Make 80 percent of your food healthy, natural, unprocessed, and clean. The remainder can be made up of a variety of things you feel like eating.

Organic and clean

To be true, some organic and pesticide-free food can be hard on the wallet, but it's preferable to pay for your food now rather than later in life when the toxins from pesticides turn up in a rash of negative health effects. The body has its own built-in detoxification system working continuously. Our problem lies in the load we heap on our bodies on a daily basis—not only from food, but from car emissions, radiation from mobile devices, deodorants, perfumes, clothes, cleaning products, gas stations, etc. But if you have the means and can afford to do so without going overboard, do your best to seek out organic produce.

How do you know if something is organic? If you don't notice clear labeling on the packaging or on a sign by the bin, you'll often find a code-number label stuck right onto the fruit or vegetable. If the produce is organic, the label will display five numbers, beginning with number nine. If the label has four numbers starting with a three or a four, the product is conventionally farmed.

Obviously, it's harder to be sure if a meal at a restaurant is organic, or when you've been invited to dine with friends. There's no need to stress, however—just remember the 80/20 rule (see above). Some situations will be out of your control, but what goes into your own refrigerator and freezer is, and that counts for a lot.

Dirty Dozen & Clean Fifteen

The Environmental Working Group (EWG) publishes a yearly review of conventionally produced foods. The products with highest pesticide residue are part of the Dirty Dozen Plus, and the ones with least pesticide residue (which are safer to eat) are called the Clean Fifteen. Here are both lists for the year 2015. (There are some variations from year to year.)

Dirty Dozen Plus

1. Apples
2. Peaches
3. Nectarines
4. Strawberries
5. Grapes
6. Celery
7. Spinach
8. Sweet bell peppers
9. Cucumber
10. Cherry tomatoes
11. Snap peas (imported)
12. Potatoes
13. Hot peppers
14. Kale/collard greens

Clean Fifteen

1. Avocados
2. Corn
3. Pineapples
4. Cabbages
5. Sugar snap peas (frozen)
6. Onions
7. Asparagus
8. Mangoes
9. Papaya
10. Kiwi
11. Eggplant
12. Grapefruit
13. Cantaloupe
14. Cauliflower
15. Sweet potatoes

Seasonal and locally raised

Nature follows certain cycles. Humans are part of nature, and so must adapt to natural, seasonal changes. This means more than hauling the winter jacket out of storage in November; it also means grocery shopping for food that is in season wherever you happen to live. These seasonal menus are comprised of food that is usually more flavorful, nutritious, and fresher than the food you would eat if you didn't follow nature's natural cycles.

When you choose to shop for locally produced, seasonal food, you also support the local economy, and reduce the energy expenditure needed for the production and transportation of food. Find out where your food comes from, and choose local food as often as possible. If you have long-standing Swedish roots, perhaps you shouldn't eat several mangoes a day. Blueberries and apples are better choices, since they are native to Sweden. Of course you can eat mangoes too, but your body is more suited to produce that grows in the Nordic countries. It makes sense, doesn't it?

Nutrition as highest priority

Nutrition should be our highest priority. We must begin to recognize that food is fuel for our bodies. We have to fill our bodies with the right kind of fuel to make it move more efficiently, not less. How often have you experienced a post-noon slump at work after a heavy lunch, when you needed at least an hour to get going again? Or eaten a bag of candy late at night, only to feel bloated the next day?

We were not designed to survive on processed foods that the body doesn't recognize. We're meant to eat living food loaded with vitamins, minerals, and enzymes. We must eat wholesome food to give us energy, strength, and harmony.

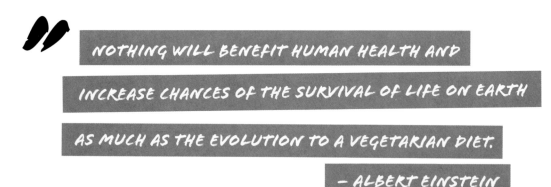

"NOTHING WILL BENEFIT HUMAN HEALTH AND INCREASE CHANCES OF THE SURVIVAL OF LIFE ON EARTH AS MUCH AS THE EVOLUTION TO A VEGETARIAN DIET.

— ALBERT EINSTEIN

PERSONAL EATING HABITS

Different foods suit different people, but I'm sure there are certain things we all should eat more or less of. These few ground rules apply to all of us: eat clean, unprocessed, seasonal, locally raised and/or farmed, organic, and green, whenever possible.

Your food choices should reflect your own needs. In order to navigate the grocery store's aisles it's important to start listening to your inner compass. What is your body telling you? How does it react to different ingredients? Do you get bloated if you eat gluten, or does your digestion remain unaffected? Do you feel tired, or energized, after a meal of pasta? Do you need a daily green smoothie to start the day off right? What does your body require, exactly, for optimal balance? If you don't quite know the answer to these questions, it's time you started paying attention; your body sends clear signals when it likes or doesn't like a certain kind of food. Often the problem is that we can't be bothered to listen, but we have to stop ignoring these signals. In my case, for instance, my stomach gets bloated, my skin breaks out, and my temper and energy levels plummet when I eat sugar. My body is very clear about when it is unhappy with my choices. This happens also with gluten, lactose, and certain other ingredients, not just sugar.

How often have you continued to eat long after your body has been satiated? Have you ever had a stomachache after eating a big steak? Have you ever added a bit of cream to a fruit dessert, even though you know the lactose would upset your stomach? Or, maybe you've felt wonderful after eating a delicious summer salad? This is feedback your body is sending you every day, so you have to become tuned in to it!

You should eat what your body needs for optimal health. Quit following your girl-friend's diet, or indulging in your mother's traditional cooking, if neither of them work for you. What do you need to feel good? Which food or ingredients create harmony within your body?

We need to be open-minded to welcome change that will improve our quality of life! Becoming healthy is a journey, and we learn how to eat while we're on it. New studies and news stories about food are constantly being published, so it's important to be open to healthier alternatives. Perhaps in five years' time your needs will be completely different. Try not to get stuck in rigid categories; instead, pick out the parts of each that work best for you. We all have to try to figure out what fits our own body. A few years ago, a worldwide research study was conducted on the longest living people. It concluded that they all ate differently from each other, but shared two common denominators: they all ate lots of vegetables, and everyone ate good fats. For that reason, all recipes in this program are full of vegetables and good fats, which will help calm your sugar cravings. Since we also want to live as long as possible, why not take a page from the books of the inhabitants of the Greek island, Ikaria, or the Japanese in Okinawa? Let go of the quick-fix mentality, and create new, healthy routines in your life instead.

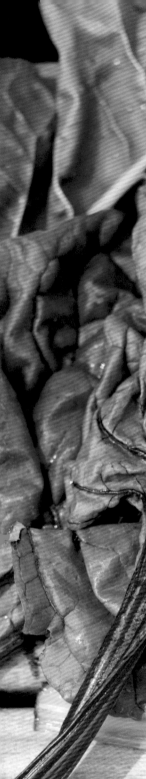

12 Start-Up Tips

1. Decrease your consumption of fruit. Eat one or two pieces of fruit a day.
2. Eat fruit that is native to your country; in Sweden, good examples would be berries and apples. Choose fruits that are in season.
3. Drink eight glasses of water a day. Water helps with digestion and cleanses the body.
4. Fifteen minutes before breakfast, drink a glass of lukewarm water with some freshly squeezed lemon juice. This is to cleanse the liver and reset the pH level.
5. Eat a fat and protein-rich snack in the afternoon to stabilize your blood sugar and prevent dips in energy before dinner.
6. Take probiotics daily to promote a healthy balance of gut bacteria.
7. Increase your intake of green vegetables. They help to calm sugar cravings, and give your body a boost of nutrients.
8. Eat regularly, about every three hours. Listen to your body; wait a while if you're not hungry after three hours, or eat a bit earlier if you are.
9. Deal with your emotions by keeping a journal. Jotting down your feelings on paper can give you some time to reflect.
10. Have fun! Don't take this process so seriously. Keep it light and enjoy the journey! Post pictures of your meals on Instagram; share your recipes with friends; or invite your family to a flavorful and healthy meal.
11. Begin each day with a nutritious breakfast; set the right tone for the day early in the morning.
12. Focus on all the food you can enjoy, instead of mulling over what you have to take a pass at. Look forward to each meal.

Find balance on your plate

I know life isn't always a walk in the park, and that goes for food choices, too. That's why I believe in making the best of each situation, and of each meal. Let go of perfectionism, and strive for realistic goals. Try to make the majority of your meals healthy and nutritious, and allow yourself to take a break now and then. Perhaps you're on a trip to Rome and the menu in front of you lists wonderful pasta dishes; or you're sitting on a dock in the sun, enjoying a big ice-cream cone. It's okay to have a little of what you love from time to time.

It's also important to thoroughly enjoy everything and to let go of feelings of guilt, which typically rear their ugly heads after an indulgence: "I should only have eaten one. How many calories are there in chocolate muffins anyway?" or "This will show up on the scale, and I really hope it was worth it." This is a common problem we encounter when we feel a loss of control, following dependency. This is why it's important to become aware

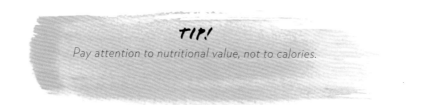

TIP!

Pay attention to nutritional value, not to calories.

of the energy behind each meal and ask ourselves if the foods we consume cause joy or stress. Behind those feelings lie the answers.

Listen to your body's hunger signals

Some people are so driven by their hunger signals that they have to answer them immediately, while others can easily ignore their belly's rumblings. It's very easy to overlook the signals and become ravenous—all it takes is a meeting that runs over, or a shopping spree with your best friend. However, your gut doesn't care one bit about the long checkout line at the store, or that your boss was rambling on (yaaaawn). Planning is in order here! I repeat: Planning. Your body has to be able to depend on you to avoid switching to starvation mode; it wants to let your metabolism get on with its work and to keep your blood glucose levels steady. However, if your body feels you're off doing your own thing and ignoring it, it will demand something sweet, and sooner rather than later. We need to avoid this situation.

I recommend that you eat something every three hours to avoid dips in blood sugar levels. Maybe you can't wait that long, so listen to your body—only you can tell. But try not to wait longer than four hours. Also, monitor how late in the day you eat—try to avoid eating past 8 p.m., or two hours before your regular bedtime. Do your best! There will always be days when this doesn't fit in, and that is perfectly okay. Choose a gentle approach, without punishment. Your digestive system will start cleaning out the intestines in the evening and will need to recover properly for optimal function. Our ancestors didn't eat once night had fallen; they also got up much earlier in the morning and went to bed much earlier in the evening.

I have planned out the next three weeks for you, but it's imperative that you turn planning into a habit once this program comes to an end. Don't forget that we want to create a lifestyle, and that will take a bit of work and energy before it becomes second nature.

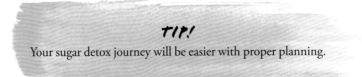

TIP!
Your sugar detox journey will be easier with proper planning.

THREE POTENTIAL PITFALLS

pH level

The pH is the measure of hydrogen-ion concentration in the body, and it tells us whether the body is alkaline or acidic. Too many acidic foods can lead to illness later in life because an acidic body robs the skeleton of minerals. This is not a good thing, especially for women, since it can increase the risk of osteoporosis.

How do you restore your pH level? All food we consume has a pH level, which in turn affects our blood's value. Even other factors—stress, for example—can cause the body to turn acidic. Your aim should be for 70 percent alkaline and 30 percent acidic foods.

ALKALINE FOODS

Spinach, broccoli, cauliflower, Brussels sprouts, carrots, cucumbers, lemons, onions, avocados, sweet potatoes, blueberries, kiwi fruit, dates, sweet almonds, artichokes, and seaweed.

ACIDIC FOODS

Refined white sugar, dairy products, alcohol, soft drinks, pasta, chocolate, vinegar, peanuts, white bread, coffee, fruit juice, eggs, fish, soy milk, artificial sweeteners, and brown rice.

Inflammation

Most inflammatory diseases begin in the gut via an autoimmune reaction and an overloaded immune system. This is not surprising, considering that 80 percent of the immune system is located in the gastrointestinal tract. Inflammation can cause, among other things: arthritis, coronary heart disease, psoriasis, cancer, allergies, and Alzheimer's disease. We eat many processed and pesticide-laden foods these days, along with huge amounts of sugar, lactose, and gluten, all of which affect the digestive system and cause imbalance. We have to rethink our habits! Start by eating organic and clean foods, which the body can recognize and use to the fullest—foods that give the body a much-needed boost of nutrients.

Food isn't the only cause of inflammation; lifestyle is another. Factors such as stress, too much or too little exercise, and bad sleeping habits can contribute to inflammatory responses in the form of asthma, eczema, allergies, and gastrointestinal illness.

The human gut harbors approximately 10,000 different types of bacteria, some of them beneficial, others not so much. We need about 80 percent "beneficial" intestinal bacteria for optimal health. You can add in the right ones by eating a daily dose of probiotics, which can be found in yogurt as well as in fermented foods like sauerkraut. You can also get probiotics through tablets and capsules—preferably taken in the mornings about fifteen minutes before breakfast. Probiotics also aid in digesting food, creating balanced intestinal flora, and strengthening the immune system.

Gluten

Gluten is a protein that is found in grains such as wheat, barley, and rye. It provides elasticity to dough, helping it to rise, retain its shape, and achieve the right consistency. Gluten can also act as an irritant on the mucous membrane and damage the lining of the small intestine, preventing the uptake of nutrients such as vitamins A, D, E, and K.

You can be affected by gluten even if you don't have a known sensitivity to it. Avoid all processed, nutrient-poor foods such as white bread and pasta, and exchange white carbohydrates for living, green produce. All the recipes in this three-week program are gluten-free.

If you don't know that you have a sensitivity to gluten, test first by removing gluten from your diet for a few weeks, and keep an eye on how you feel. How is your gut? How are your energy levels and mental alertness? Then reintroduce gluten into your meals for a few days and gauge how your body reacts.

PERSONAL AND CLEAN

To sum it up, there isn't one single diet that is optimal for everyone, as we're all different people with different needs. Find out what suits you and your body best, and then aim to always eat as unprocessed, clean, and organic as possible.

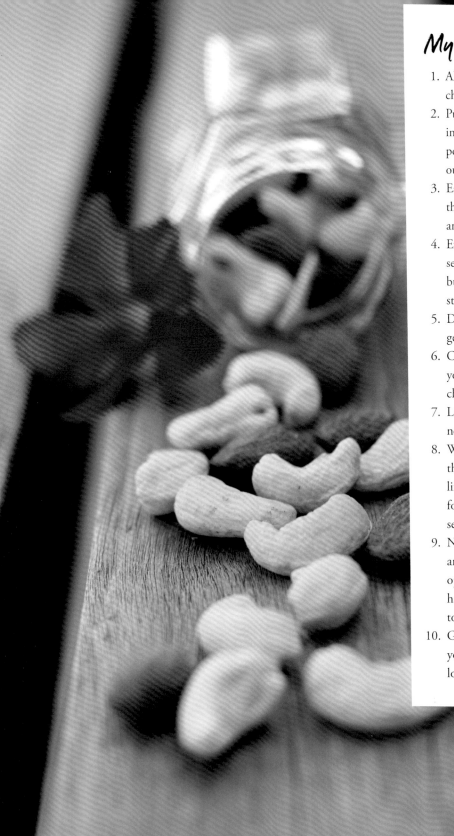

My top 10 health tips!

1. Always aim to do your best when choosing food and occasion.
2. Put an end to negative thoughts immediately, and say something positive instead. Whatever you send out will come back to you!
3. Eat a protein and fat-rich snack in the afternoon to keep your energy up and steady.
4. Experience food with all of your senses. Satisfy your eyes, your taste buds, your nose, as well as your stomach when you eat.
5. Drink a glass of water as soon as you get up in the morning.
6. Concentrate on adding good food to your diet, instead of removing bad choices.
7. Listen to your body's signals and needs—it knows its requirements best.
8. Weight is not the most important thing, so don't let the scales run your life and emotions. Eat wholesome food, and your weight will reach its set point naturally.
9. New studies about food and health are constantly coming out. Keep an open mind about change. Nobody has all the answers, and we learn together along the way.
10. Get moving. Find some exercise that you like to do. Exercise because you love your body.

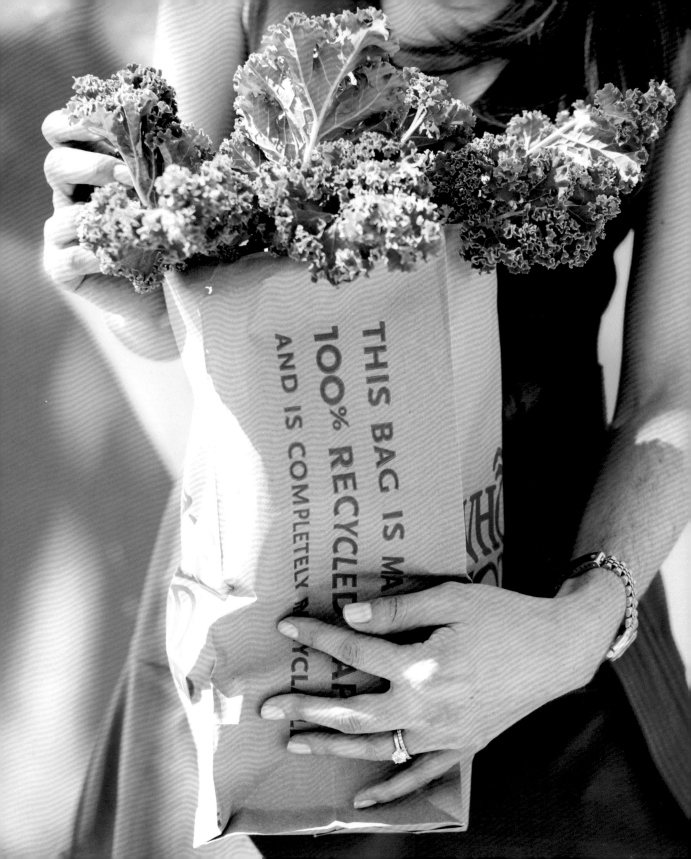

CHAPTER 4

Your Sugar Detox Program

HERE IT IS—THE PROGRAM THAT WILL SHOW YOU HOW TO STOP EATING SUGAR FOR THREE WEEKS. INCLUDED ARE RECIPE PLANS, SHOPPING LISTS FOR EACH OF THE WEEKS, AND EXERCISES IN CREATING YOUR OWN AFFIRMATIONS AND MINDFUL EATING. IT'S EVERYTHING YOU'LL NEED TO MAKE THIS SUGAR DETOX AS SIMPLE AND ENJOYABLE AS POSSIBLE!

IN THREE WEEKS YOU WILL HAVE A NEW RELATIONSHIP WITH SUGAR. A relationship that is calm, free, and easy. You'll be able to make food choices based on intuition and real hunger, instead of letting sugar control your options. You don't need to avoid sugar forever, only for twenty-one days. That's enough time to break the habit and reset your body. First up is the week of preparation, when you'll reduce your intake of sugar and clear out all sugar from your kitchen. The following weeks are as follows: Detox Week, Nutrition Week, and Final Week. There's a menu for each week (including a shopping list), adapted for the week you're currently in and covering all the items you'll need.

This is not a restrictive diet; it is, however, a time devoted to respect. Are you ready to fortify your body? To give up your sugar habit? To find the motivation, and to quiet the negative inner chatter that doesn't believe you can do this? Of course you can create a healthy relationship with sugar! Don't listen to the silliness in your head. After all, you're reading this book, aren't you? There's a reason why it's in your hands at this very moment. You are ready. You'll make it. Ditch that can of soda sitting on your desk right now and pour yourself a mug of warm lemon water. It's sugar detox time!

12 BENEFITS OF CUTTING BACK ON SUGAR

1. Steady energy levels
2. Clearer and more luminous skin
3. Less risk of developing certain diseases
4. Mental clarity
5. Freedom from sugar's hold
6. Better body image
7. Clearer hunger signals
8. Healthier connection to your emotions
9. Increased nutritional boost for the body
10. Better balance in life
11. Steady blood glucose levels
12. Healthier and lighter body

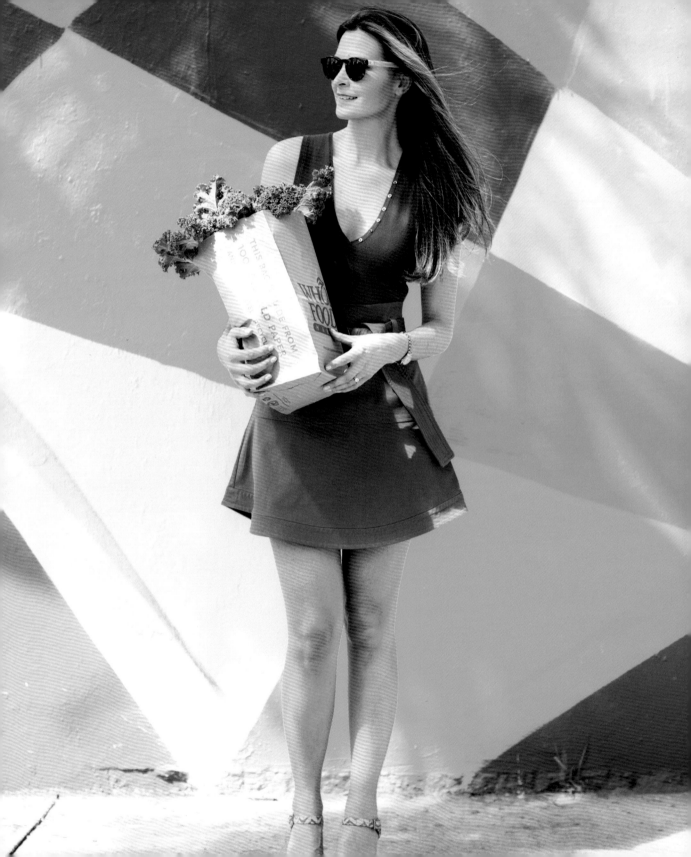

BEFORE YOU BEGIN

Planning and preparation

How many times have you come home, exhausted after a long day at work, only to throw together a boring, quick-fix dinner? Perhaps you poured yourself a bowl of cereal and milk, or picked at your kids' sausage and pasta dinner? Well, we're changing all that. Planning is the key to a successful sugar detox; you must prepare ahead for each week. The menu is already set, but you'll need to shop for groceries so everything is in place when you stumble through the door after work.

Most of my dinners can be made in less than thirty minutes, some even less! Breakfast recipes require five to ten minutes; lunch is a snap since it's made up of leftovers from dinner the night before. You only need to cook one meal per day. If you still have more leftovers, you can store them in the freezer. The program's recipes are suitable for everybody; the ingredients were selected to agree with most people. This is not a diet—you don't have to prepare separate meals for the rest of your family, but you can always add a piece of fish or grass-fed beef if someone requests it. Maybe a piece of salmon with the nori rolls, or a slice of ham with the Mediterranean plate? You can also try to serve the program's menu as is. Who knows, maybe both you and your family might end up preferring to go vegetarian.

Do buy some vitamin B_{12} tablets; B_{12} is important for strengthening the immune system, stabilizing energy levels, and improving mental acuity and cell development. You can choose from several different brands available at health food markets.

Your food should be prepared with loving care; eating is far more enjoyable when someone has put in the effort to make a meal. That's why we oftentimes have such vivid memories of food from childhood, perhaps of grandma's fresh-baked cinnamon buns or dad's spaghetti and meat sauce. But let's not start craving those things! This program will show you that lovingly prepared food can also be healthy! It's the kind of food that requires a bit of time and planning. Over the next few weeks, organize your time and set aside the hours it will take for you to succeed. You might already have all the ingredients for the recipes, or they may need to be purchased at the beginning of the week. You'll have no excuses if you have them on hand, since you won't have to waste time running to the grocery store. We want to prevent you from becoming ravenous, so if everything is prepared at home you can start cooking as soon as you're in the door after work. Keep it simple.

If you don't enjoy cooking, you'll have to think of it as a necessary evil. But who knows, perhaps this sugar detox will change your mind and you'll start to feel more comfortable in the kitchen. Don't become frustrated if things don't come out perfect; try again and you might have better luck next time around.

Don't forget to enjoy yourself! Try to have fun with this even if your brain is doing its best to convince you that it's hard. Rubbish—this is going to be so simple for you. Repeat your affirmation (see page 58) if your brain begins to play tricks on you. Make this experience educational, thrilling, loving, and fun. Let's have a good time!

Basic ingredients

Stock your kitchen cupboards with the basic ingredients and flavorful spices that you'll use throughout the program; that way you'll have no excuses for not having tasty, healthy food to eat because everything will be right there. Start by putting together a shopping list and write down everything you need to get. We'll add more items on the following pages. The following is a list of good ingredients to have on hand.

• Baking powder
• Buckwheat flour
• Dijon mustard
• Ghee (clarified butter)
• Vegetable stock
• Cold-pressed olive oil
• Coconut flour
• Coconut oil
• Almond flour
• Almond butter
• Unrefined salt, such as Himalayan or Celtic sea salt
• Spirulina powder
• Tahini paste
• Tamari soy sauce
• White wine vinegar

Spice and herb guide

Well-seasoned food provides plenty of health benefits. For example, turmeric is an anti-inflammatory, and oregano contains vitamin K, which is good for your skeletal structure. It's time to add some spice to your life!

- **Chili powder** - boosts the immune system and can lower cholesterol levels.
- **Turmeric** - calms a bloated stomach and removes toxins.
- **Ginger** - calms the intestines and is an anti-inflammatory.
- **Cinnamon** - can lessen sugar cravings while it helps regulate blood glucose levels.
- **Cardamom** - helps digestion.
- **Cumin** - can improve memory and reduce stress.
- **Oregano** - can protect against colds and calm digestive upsets.
- **Rosemary** - stimulates the immune system and improves blood flow.
- **Black pepper** - contributes intestinal health.
- **Thyme** - good for fighting cough and respiratory problems.
- **Vanilla powder** - protects the liver and is anti-inflammatory.

What shall I drink during the program?

- Water
- Lukewarm water with freshly squeezed lemon juice
- Lukewarm water with fresh mint leaves
- Tea
- Green juices
- Unsweetened nut milks
- Coconut water
- Homemade stock
- Coffee

Yes, you can stop holding your breath—you are allowed to drink coffee. It's still a good idea, however, to avoid drinking it while you're on the program so you can let your body create stable energy without going through slumps. If you must have coffee, drink one single cup per day, and without sugar, of course.

Clean out your pantry

Grab a garbage bag and start cleaning out your pantry, refrigerator, and freezer. Your kitchen can take a sugar detox. If you'd prefer not to throw out food, pass it on to friends or family. Or you can even leave a box of it with your neighbor, to be returned to you once you feel strong enough to have sugar in the home again. To avoid temptation, it's best to keep sugar out of the house for the duration of the program.

Thoroughly check the nutrition label on each item. For example, some bouillon cubes contain sugar, while others don't. Be your own health detective. Scan the list on the following page for ingredients that could contain sugar. It might surprise you to find certain items on the list, but there are lots of hidden sugars in our food.

How do you read a nutrition label?

How do you know if the items in your shopping cart contain sugar and artificial sweeteners? Hidden sugars can be found in the most surprising places. Look for the following names:

- Acesulfame-K
- Aspartame
- Cyclamate and its Na and Ca salts
- Erythritol
- Fructose
- High Fructose Corn Syrup
- Glucose
- Glucose syrup
- Invert sugar syrup
- Isomalt
- Lactitol
- Lactose
- Maltitol and maltitol syrup
- Mannitol
- Neohesperidin DC (NHDC)
- Saccharin and its Na-, K- and Ca salts
- Sucrose
- Sugars
- Sorbitol and sorbitol syrup
- Sucralose
- Thaumatin
- Xylitol

AWAY FROM YOUR KITCHEN

The most challenging part of sticking to the plan and eating healthy is when your social life gets in the way. Everything runs smoothly when you're at home and free to choose what to eat—no problems there. However, sometimes a monkey wrench gets thrown into the works.

Keep your cool when a client confirms a dinner date in the middle of the week, or when friends invite you out to lunch. You'll be fine. I have lots of tips on how to stay social while continuing to avoid sugar. Obviously, you have to continue living your life even if you're not eating sweets for the time being!

Get rid of these items

You don't have to feel that this is farewell forever, because you can reintroduce some of the following foods in reasonable amounts after you finish the program.

- Balsamic vinegar
- Bouillon (stock) cubes, if they contain sugar
- Chips
- Energy drinks
- Breakfast cereals and muesli
- Fruit
- Ready-to-eat soups
- Ready-to-eat sauces
- Ice cream
- Candy
- Honey
- Ketchup
- Concentrated juices, fruit juices, and cordials
- Fruit-based desserts
- "Light" products and artificial sweeteners
- Soda
- Pizza
- Potatoes
- Processed soy, rice, and nut milks
- Refined bread and cookies
- Raw and energy bars
- Sugar syrup
- Sweetened yogurt
- Tomato sauce, if it contains added sugar
- Dried fruit
- Vinaigrette dressing
- Refined pasta
- White rice
- Refined sugar

Dinner invitations

When you find yourself in social situations, keep listening to your body and eat what is good for you. No one else knows what goes on in your body, and how it reacts to different foods. It is your mission to learn its deeper signs and to start taking care of its needs. You can't always follow society's rules—they change constantly. You have to follow your own path, both during the three weeks of the program and thereafter. It's crazy to consume things your body can't handle, which in this case is sugar. You'll probably be able to enjoy a piece of chocolate, a cookie, or a scoop of ice cream sometime in the future without doing any damage, but at the moment it's vital that you avoid all sugars. Thankfully, it is possible to have a social life without eating sugar.

Plan. It's easier for everyone when you know what your food options are. If you get invited to dinner, maybe you get in touch with the hosts and ask what is on the menu. Then you'll be mentally prepared and won't stray from the program.

Explain your problem with sugar. If you're visiting family or friends, contact them ahead of time and let them know about the program, and why you're following it. The more you share and explain, the more understanding they'll be, and hopefully the more eager to help you stay on the plan. We hope the hosts prefer that you accept their invitation, instead of declining it because of the program.

If you have contacted the hosts and they're unsure about what to serve you, offer to bring a dish or to help them out once you're there. Make alternative suggestions. You could even email them a recipe—perhaps something from this book?

Dining in restaurants

Dining out can present some challenges, even when you're not undergoing a sugar detox. We entrust the meal's preparation to a stranger, so we don't know the quality of the ingredients, how much of them are used, or the manner in which they're cooked. But you can always find out from your servers—this is your right as a customer. When you're dealing with sugar, it's better to be safe than sorry and take a few minutes to ask some questions. As you already know, hidden sugar is everywhere, such as in balsamic vinegar, as well as stocks and sauces. Stay vigilant—especially when following the program.

- Look over the menu before you decide which restaurant to go to; many eateries offer healthy dishes these days. If you can't find an acceptable place, call the restaurant's kitchen and see if the chef is willing to make a dish especially for you. They can often sauté some vegetables or mix a salad with ingredients they already have on hand, even if it's not on the menu.
- Fish, shellfish, soup, or anything vegetable-based make the best appetizers and entrées.
- Skip the colorful cocktails and, yes—the wine. Instead, order some fresh still or sparkling water. By all means, add in some lemon, lime, or cucumber for a bit of flavor.
- Avoid white carbohydrates such as potatoes, pasta, rice, and pizza. Ask your waiter to remove the tempting bread basket from the table as soon as possible to alleviate unnecessary torment.
- Ask about the sugar content of sauces and dressings. Remember there is hidden sugar in tomato sauce, ketchup, and balsamic vinegar. Dressing is a safe bet if it's made with olive oil, vinegar, salt, and pepper—a fresh and healthy option.
- If you're still hungry and would like to eat dessert, order some cheese or a cup of tea. Omit the honey, though.

Remember what's really important here—company and friendship. Focus on conversation instead of on the sugar bombs listed on the dessert menu. Chocolate fondue is overrated, right? All joking aside, it is divine, but it's even better to rid yourself of your sensitivity to sugar—I promise.

What about the coffee break?

If you can resist rushing up to the counter to order something while the aroma of fresh-baked pastries lingers in the air, then by all means enjoy a cup of coffee in a café. However, if that first glimpse of torte brings on an episode of stress and anxiety, stay clear of coffee shops while you follow the program. You can give it a shot to see how you feel. Steel yourself mentally before going in, and only order what you have decided on.

If you eat something beforehand, you won't be as tempted by all the things on display, and you'll just order a beverage. You can also take a coffee break at home or at a friend's place. Then you'll have more options to choose from:

- A vegetable smoothie or juice without fruit
- Chai tea made from oat, almond, or coconut milk
- Nuts mixed with cinnamon, vanilla, and salt
- Oven-roasted nuts, seeds, coconut flakes, and spice mix
- Home-baked sugar-free muffins
- Home-baked bread (see page 86) with different varieties of nut butters, mashed avocado with lemon and salt, sliced tomato with olive oil and pepper, or cheese with bell pepper or cucumber.

ON THE GO TIPS!

- **Keep your eye on the prize.** Focus on your goal and what is important for you. Is it to eat a pastry when having a coffee with a friend, or lose your sugar sensitivity?
- **Plan your next step.** If you know you're going to be out and about for hours, make sure to stash some nuts in your bag, or find out where you can buy a quick and healthy snack in town.
- **Respect yourself.** You don't have to eat sweets just because others do it.
- **Find inner strength so you can say no.** You are worth so much more than the fleeting sensation of refined sugar and all its aftereffects.
- **Fill your bag with snacks that contain good fats and protein.** That way you have something easy to grab for when you need a boost of energy.
- **Tell your companions about the program you're following before you order food.** You're responsible for your own order; nobody should try to tempt you with sweets.
- **Choose the best option.** Do the best you can—that's all you can do in every situation. Work-related travel can be extra problematic, but try to plan things in advance and make the best of the situation.
- **Enjoy some popcorn made with coconut oil while cozying up on the sofa with the family on Friday night.** You needn't feel excluded because they pick at the contents of the candy dish. You never know, though, they might want to join you for some popcorn instead!

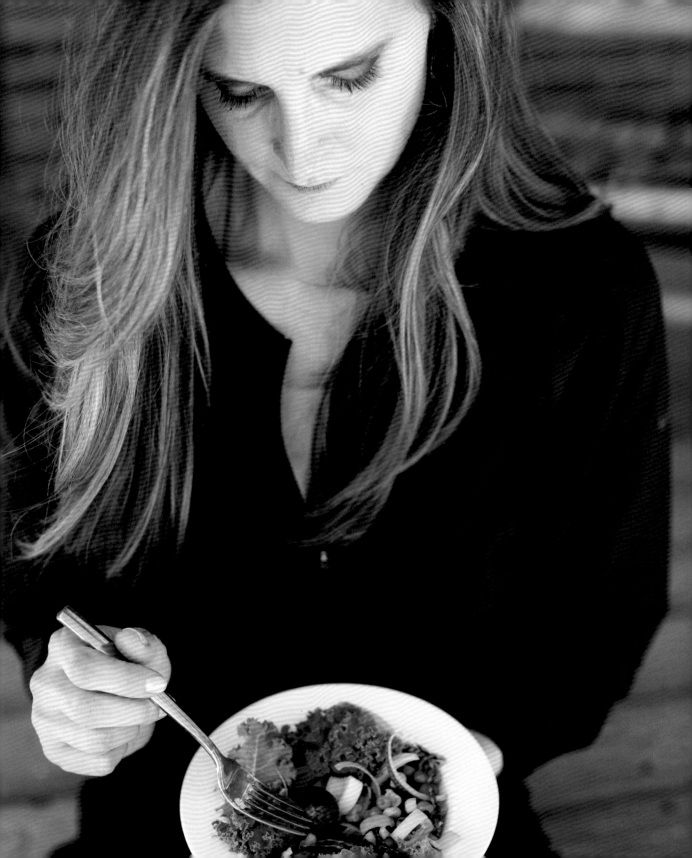

MINDFUL EATING

It's important to pay attention to each bite you eat, because if you're not mindful at the dinner table you'll miss the entire experience. You won't taste the flavors if your gaze is stuck on the TV screen instead of on your plate; you'll miss the delicious aromas wafting from the stove while you're busy chatting on the phone. Consequently, you'll remain unsatisfied and hungry after such a meal, so you'll go back to the kitchen to find something more "fun" to eat—something to lighten your everyday boredom. Mindful eating, however, can mitigate this problem.

Now you will begin to taste, smell, notice, and enjoy your food. You will call on all your senses when you eat for a richer experience. This will leave you content when you put down your knife and fork and swallow the last bite. You're going to feel satisfied when you finish a meal. Use these mindful eating tips as often as possible, especially when eating at home.

EXERCISE: MINDFUL EATING

Set a beautiful table: Set the table in the kitchen or in the dining room. Include a place mat, a plate, some flatware, a glass, and a napkin. Light a candle to create a harmonious atmosphere. Don't eat in the living room if you don't normally eat your meals in there.

Be present: Turn off all electronic devices, and put away anything that might distract you during your meal such as cell phones, newspapers, books, work reports, radio, TV, and computers.

Observe: Serve your meal. Look at the food. Picture that this will actually become part of your body—it's absolutely fascinating.

Smell: Inhale deeply through your nose to catch all the aromas.

Be grateful: Give thanks to the food for all its nourishment and energy.

Taste: Take a bite and chew it deliberately. Chew every mouthful at least twenty times—your digestive system will thank you. Feel and experience the flavors and textures.

Pause: Put down your fork between bites. Continue to look, smell, and taste your food throughout the meal.

POSITIVE AFFIRMATIONS

Do you have a negative inner voice that often tries to sabotage you? Does it tend to get louder when things finally start looking up for you? This journey is also about silencing that nasty chatter, and listening to your heart and to your feelings. There is no truth in a voice that is hell-bent on undermining you. It is a false messenger. You are enough—you are perfect just the way you are. You can live your life without sugar controlling your choices and your temper. We will begin to listen to that loving inner voice. You will let it guide you to respect your body through the healthy food choices you make.

Positive thoughts bring about positive results. The energy you send out will come back to you. This is the law of attraction that I mentioned in the introduction. If you think this is mere hocus-pocus, just try it and see what happens. Give it a chance!

EXERCISE: CREATE YOUR POSITIVE AFFIRMATION

A self-created positive affirmation can nudge you in the right direction—a helpful expression that can become your slogan for the upcoming weeks. You can use it as a mantra when the going gets tough, so it will keep you on the straight and narrow. You can post it on your bedroom wall, or make it background of your cell phone. Repeat your positive affirmation as often as you feel the need, and remind yourself what you're trying to achieve by going through this program. What is your personal goal?

Write your positive affirmation in the present tense and avoid negative words such as *not*. You can create your own, or choose from my examples:

- I am free from my sugar addiction
- I eat clean foods that help every cell in my body
- It's easy to let go of sugar and to eat healthily
- I respect my body, and choose the right kind of food
- I have a normal relationship with food
- I eat healthily and listen to my body
- I live a sugar-free life
- I can get rid of my addiction to sugar
- I am able to pass up sugar for three weeks
- I choose to respect myself today
- I am strong enough to cope with the sugar detox program

Send out your positive affirmation energy by telling a friend or a family member, or post it on Instagram with the hashtag **#sugardetox**. I'm behind you all the way. We should all help each other with encouraging words via social media. Use today's resources to give and receive help.

EMOTIONS BEHIND THE SUGAR

Just as there are two sides to every coin, there are also two sides to sugar dependency. One is connected to the chemical reactions that take place in the body, a topic we covered earlier in this book. The other side concerns your feelings—how you use sugar to calm them, to cope with them, to comfort, or ignore them. Perhaps you haven't made the connection before? Have you ever run down and bought a sweetened chai latte to relieve your boredom at work? Have you felt lonely, only to keep company with a pint of Ben & Jerry's? Have you looked for love in a coffee shop, but left the premises with two pastries in your belly instead? We're often not aware of our behavior, or know exactly what is happening, but find an action difficult to stop once it has begun. We all have our own reasons and emotions steering our behavior around food. Feelings that want to be heard. Feelings that want to lead us. But we choose to ignore them and demand that sugar fix instead, for protection or help. But you won't find solutions or answers to your problems in a cookie. Sugar is the worst weapon you can use because it only creates more conflict within you.

The objective is to give yourself time and space to experience your feelings. They carry important messages. You have to work through your feelings to be able to let go of them—there is no way to avoid them. As I've said, there are answers to much bigger questions hiding behind your feelings.

How often do you use food to avoid dealing with feelings? The time has come to look inward. Life will be so much easier once you learn to feel and listen to your heart—your body's own GPS.

Live fully

Food tends to play a major role in our lives. Many of us think constantly about our next meal—what we can allow ourselves to indulge in, or what we are going to offer to our dinner guests next week. Maybe you're already planning your Christmas feast. While it is important to plan, we also have to back away a little. We should eat to live, and not live to eat. You have the same amount of hours at your disposal as the rest of us each morning, so how do you choose to spend the time? Do you leave enough time for things you love? Try your best to live fully each day. There are many more things that your inner self would like to do other than eating chocolate; trust me, I've been there. You're now going to start to do what makes you happy, and not use sugar as a meager substitute for that joy.

EXERCISE: FIND YOUR REAL SOURCES OF JOY

Make a list of what you can do instead of turning to candy. It's important that you focus on meaningful activities that bring you moments of joy, like a walk in the woods, listening to stimulating music, or reading the latest best seller.

TIPS FOR DEALING WITH SUGAR CRAVINGS

- Drink a glass of water
- Get out of the kitchen for 10 minutes
- Go for a walk
- Listen to calming music, or meditate
- Drink a green juice or a smoothie
- Eat a snack containing protein and good fats
- Be present in the moment—recognize the emotions behind the craving
- Have a cup of tea or lukewarm lemon water
- Brush your teeth
- Remind yourself of your goal, and repeat your positive affirmation

Prep week

This is prep week, and it's all about getting ready for the program. It's important to be ready for the upcoming weeks! The rest of the program will be much easier if you don't shock your body, but remove sugar little by little, and switch it out for healthier options.

Eat your meals as you normally would, while limiting your intake of refined and processed sugar. Try to avoid white sugar, candy, chocolate,

Top 20 ingredients that appease sugar cravings

Stock your pantry with these excellent ingredients and let them help you.

1. **Chia seeds**
2. **Spirulina**
3. **Coconut oil**
4. **Sweet almonds**
5. **Ground flaxseed**
6. **Walnuts**
7. **Chlorella**
8. **Bee pollen**
9. **Avocado**
10. **Quinoa**
11. **Garlic**
12. **Lemon**
13. **Sprouts**
14. **Spinach**
15. **Broccoli**
16. **Olive oil**
17. **Unrefined salt**
18. **Nutritional yeast**
19. **Poppy seeds**
20. **Salmon**

pastries, cookies, sodas, agave syrup, concentrated juice, and ice cream. You can still eat foods such as fruit, berries, honey, and dates, all of which contain natural sugars. But reduce these amounts here too, as it will make the transition to the three-week program much easier on you.

Are you ready to purge your pantry and plan the upcoming weeks? To turn negative thoughts into positive affirmations? Good, let's get this show on the road!

Week 1: Detox week

Here is where you begin the program proper. How do you feel? I hope you feel strong, charged up, and excited. Just let go of any anxiety—you're going to do a great job! Believe me, it's easier than you think—I know because I have been down this road myself, and have succeeded in cutting my bind to sugar.

This is called detox week because it's now out with the old. We're concentrating on letting go of old habits regarding sugar and negative feelings. You're going to clean out your body to make room for optimal health, balance, and a natural way of living. The food is vegetarian, gluten-free, and packed with nutrient-rich vegetables, satisfying protein, and good fats.

You'll find the shopping list for this week's recipes on the next page. The next chapter features the recipes on pages 78–123.

Meal plan

Monday
Breakfast: Protein muesli with creamy yogurt
Lunch: Vegetarian nori rolls with tamari sauce
Dinner: Gluten-free cauliflower pizza

Tuesday
Breakfast: Green herbed omelet
Lunch: Gluten-free cauliflower pizza
Snack: Roasted rosemary almonds
Dinner: Butternut squash soup with roasted squash seeds

Wednesday

Breakfast: Lovely green smoothie

Lunch: Butternut squash soup with roasted squash seeds

Snack: Edamame dip with vegetable sticks

Dinner: Quinoa pancakes with green bean "fries"

Thursday

Breakfast: Power loaf with avocado

Lunch: Quinoa pancakes with green bean "fries"

Snack: Juicy green booster

Dinner: Mediterranean plate

Friday

Breakfast: Protein muesli with creamy yogurt

Lunch: Mediterranean plate

Snack: Coconut chia seed pudding

Dinner: Lettuce tacos and cauliflower rice with chili & guacamole

Saturday

Breakfast: Coconut pancakes with ricotta topping

Lunch: Lettuce tacos and cauliflower rice with chili & guacamole

Snack: Roasted rosemary almonds

Dinner: Baked sweet potato with ginger stuffing

Sunday

Breakfast: Protein muesli with creamy yogurt

Lunch: Baked sweet potato with ginger stuffing

Snack: Coconut chia seed pudding

Dinner: Colorful quinoa bowl

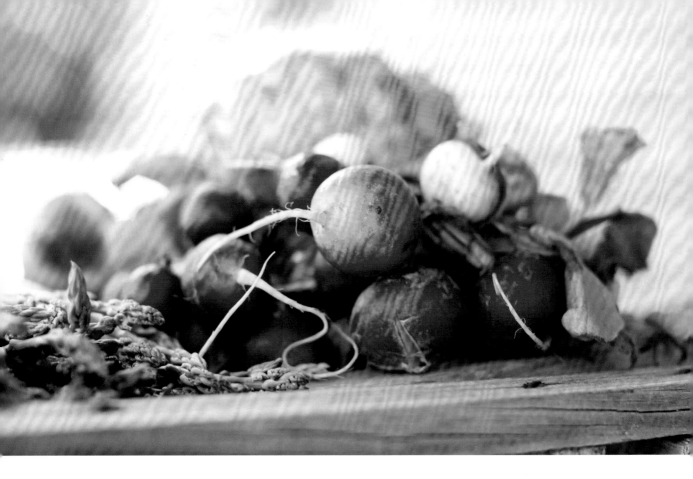

Week 1: Detoxing week

You will find all you need for this week's recipes under the headings Dairy & Eggs, Dry Ingredients & Oils, and Vegetables. Use your phone to take a picture of the list, because we're going shopping. Also, take a picture of your grocery cart before paying, and post it to Instagram with the hashtag #sugardetox so we can help each other. It's such a great feeling to leave the grocery store with so many healthy treats!

You'll be buying more food during the first week, since you'll be replenishing your stock of basic ingredients. This week you'll also need to stock your home with unrefined salt, black pepper, ground cinnamon, ground cardamom, dried oregano, dried thyme, chili powder, vanilla powder, dried rosemary, baking powder, olive oil, coconut oil, white wine vinegar, tahini, tamari, vegetable stock cubes, coconut flour, spirulina powder, almond butter, and buckwheat flour. Double-check to see if you already have some of those ingredients in your pantry.

Week 1: Shopping List

Dairy & Eggs
1 cup (2¼ dl) ricotta cheese
¾ cup (2 dl) Parmesan cheese
12 large eggs
9½ tbsp feta cheese
2½ cups (6 dl) cups Greek or Russian yogurt
¾ cup (2 dl) mozzarella cheese, grated

Dry Ingredients & Oils
3¼ cups (7½ dl) sweet almonds
1¼ cups (2½ dl) walnuts
6 tbsp chia seeds
2½ tsp poppy seeds
¼ cup (½ dl) sesame seeds
1 tsp hemp seeds
1 tsp ground flaxseed
2¾ cups (6½ dl) coconut water
1¼ cups (3 dl) almond milk
¼ cup (½ dl) tomato sauce, unsweetened
2 cups (4½ dl) coconut flakes
1 tbsp capers
1¼ cups (3 dl) chickpeas, cooked
5¼ oz (150 gr) white beans
10 olives, pitted
4½ cups (10½ dl) quinoa, cooked
4 sheets nori

Vegetables
5½ avocados
5 lemons
½ lime
2 garlic cloves
2 sweet potatoes
2¾ inch (7 cm) fresh ginger
1 butternut squash
7 carrots
3 beets
4 large lettuce leaves
1½ lbs (650 g) spinach
1⅛ lbs (500 g) kale
8¾ oz (250 g) green beans
12½ oz (350 g) edamame or peas
1 zucchini
¾ cup (2 dl) broccoli
1½ tomatoes
3 celery stalks
4 hothouse (English) cucumbers
10 Brussels sprouts
1¼ cauliflower
½ yellow bell pepper
3½ oz (100 g) mushrooms
1 red onion
1 small yellow onion
fresh basil
fresh chives
fresh parsley
lemongrass

Week 2: Nutrition week

Your body is now in full detox mode. How do you feel? Now we can start focusing on everything that you are allowed to eat. This part of the program is called nutrition week because you're loading up on nutrient-packed meals that give a boost to your body. Don't get tempted by soda at work; instead, quell your bad-for-you sugar cravings with wholesome and nutritious alternatives. Keep going! You've already gone through a whole week without sugar. Congratulations! You should be proud of yourself! Imagine telling someone that you've made it through the entire sugar detox program. Keep at it, Sugar Detox Guru! This week includes some new recipes that you haven't had a chance to sample yet.

You'll find the shopping list on the next page, and the recipes in the next chapter, pages 78–123.

Meal plan

Monday

Breakfast: Lovely green smoothie
Lunch: Colorful quinoa bowl
Snack: Coconut chia seed pudding
Dinner: Root vegetable hash with spinach

Tuesday

Breakfast: Power loaf with avocado
Lunch: Root vegetable hash with spinach
Snack: Avocado with poppy seeds and lemon
Dinner: Brussels sprout salad with Parmesan cheese and garlicky mushrooms

Wednesday

Breakfast: Green herb omelet
Lunch: Brussels sprout salad with Parmesan cheese and garlicky mushrooms
Snack: Edamame dip with vegetable sticks
Dinner: Spicy oven-roasted eggplant

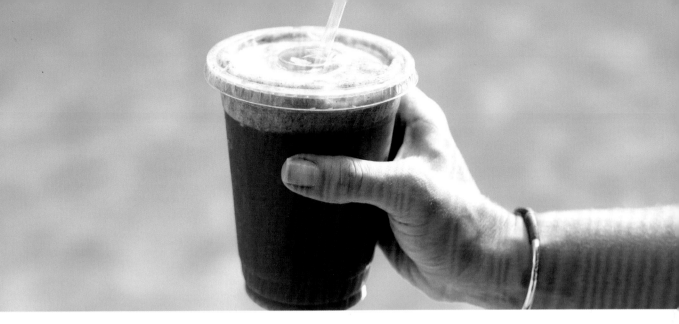

Thursday

Breakfast: Lovely green smoothie

Lunch: Spicy oven-roasted eggplant

Snack: Roasted rosemary almonds

Dinner: Chickpea salad with basil pesto

Friday

Breakfast: Protein muesli with creamy yogurt

Lunch: Chickpea salad with basil pesto

Snack: Juicy green booster

Dinner: Warm lentil salad with roasted vegetables and feta cheese

Saturday

Breakfast: Green herb omelet

Lunch: Warm lentil salad with roasted vegetables and feta cheese

Snack: Avocado with poppy seeds and lemon

Dinner: Spicy red Thai curry

Sunday

Breakfast: Coconut pancakes with ricotta topping

Lunch: Spicy red Thai curry

Snack: Coconut chia seed pudding

Dinner: Artichoke with herbed ghee

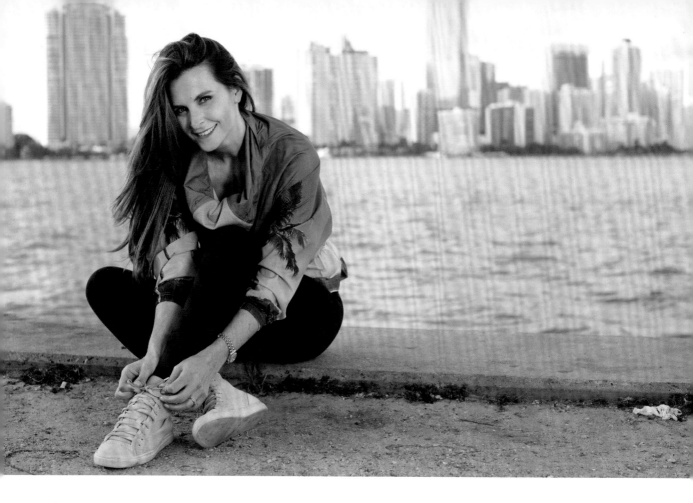

Week 2: Nutrition week

To the right you'll find all you need for this week's recipes under the headings Dairy & Eggs, Dry Ingredients & Oils, and Vegetables.

For this week you will also need unrefined salt, black pepper, ground cinnamon, chili powder, ground turmeric, vanilla powder, dried rosemary, baking powder, spirulina powder, olive oil, coconut oil, tahini, ghee, coconut flour, and Dijon mustard. These are basic ingredients, so you might already have some of them in your kitchen. If something's missing, just add it to the shopping list.

Week 2: Shopping list

Dairy & Eggs
¾ cup (2 dl) Parmesan cheese
5 large eggs
2½ oz (70 g) Parmesan cheese, grated
1 tbsp ricotta or Russian yogurt
1¼ cup (3 dl) Greek or Russian yogurt
¾ cup fresh mozzarella cheese
¾ cup (2 dl) feta cheese
1 (7 oz or 200 g) haloumi cheese

Dry Ingredients & Oils
6 tbsp chia seeds
2 tsp hemp seeds
¼ cup (½ dl) pine nuts
20 raw sweet almonds
1 can (14¼ oz or 400 ml) coconut milk
3½ cups (8 dl) coconut water
2 cups (5 dl) almond milk
1½ tsp red curry paste
1 tbsp coconut flakes
1¾ cups (4 dl) chick peas
1¼ cups (3 dl) green lentils

Vegetables
5 garlic cloves
1 red onion
2 yellow onions

1½ inch (4 cm) fresh ginger
1½ bunch broccoli
2 zucchinis
2 red bell peppers
7 carrots
2 sweet potatoes
2 tomatoes
½ cup (1 dl) sweet peas
1 lb (450 g) mushrooms
½ lime
2½ avocados
2½ lemons
30 Brussels sprouts
1¼ lbs (600 g) spinach
½ lb (250 g) kale
2 stalks celery
1½ hothouse (English) cucumbers
8 radishes
2 artichokes
2 eggplants
10 asparagus spears
¼ cup (½ dl) parsley
1 bunch basil
fresh chives
1 container sprouts, any kind
12½ oz (350 g) edamame

Week 3: Final week

You're entering the last week—the homestretch! Do you feel any different? You have detoxed from sugar for two weeks now, and I can promise you that your body is thanking you. This week we're adding a whole new breakfast recipe. You can also begin to think about how you want to eat once the program is over. The last chapter contains tips on how to continue, but it's important that you feel what is right for you.

This is the final week. Imagine the feeling of not having had any sugar for three weeks. I know you can, and that you want to reach this goal. This is it! Make way for healthier, more nutritious, and energy-packed food!

You'll find the shopping list on the next page, and the recipes in the next chapter, pages 78–123.

Meal plan

Monday
Breakfast: Lovely green smoothie
Lunch: Artichoke with herbed ghee
Snack: Avocado with poppy seeds and lemon
Dinner: Spicy oven-roasted eggplant

Tuesday
Breakfast: Protein muesli with creamy yogurt
Lunch: Spicy oven-roasted eggplant
Snack: Coconut chia seed pudding
Dinner: Vegetarian nori rolls with tamari sauce

Wednesday
Breakfast: Green herb omelet
Lunch: Vegetarian nori rolls with tamari sauce
Snack: Roasted rosemary almonds
Dinner: Butternut squash soup with roasted squash seeds

Thursday
Breakfast: Power loaf with avocado
Lunch: Butternut squash soup with roasted squash seeds

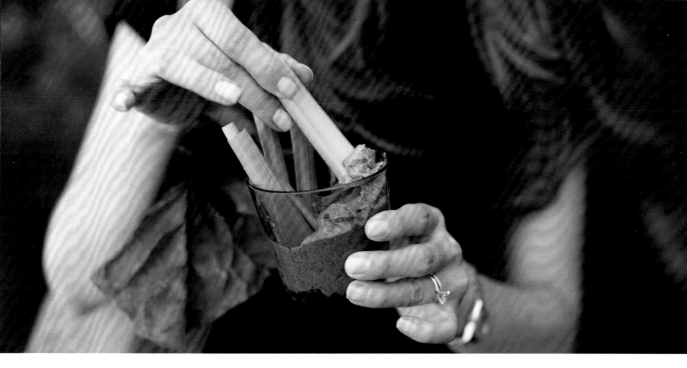

Snack: Edamame dip with vegetable sticks
Dinner: Savory corn frittata

Friday

Breakfast: Lovely green smoothie
Lunch: Savory corn frittata
Snack: Juice green booster
Dinner: Mediterranean plate

Saturday

Breakfast: Healthy scrambled eggs
Lunch: Mediterranean plate
Snack: Roasted rosemary almonds
Dinner: Gluten-free cauliflower pizza

Sunday

Breakfast: Coconut pancakes with ricotta topping
Lunch: Gluten-free cauliflower pizza
Snack: Juicy green booster
Dinner: Warm lentil salad with roasted vegetables and feta cheese

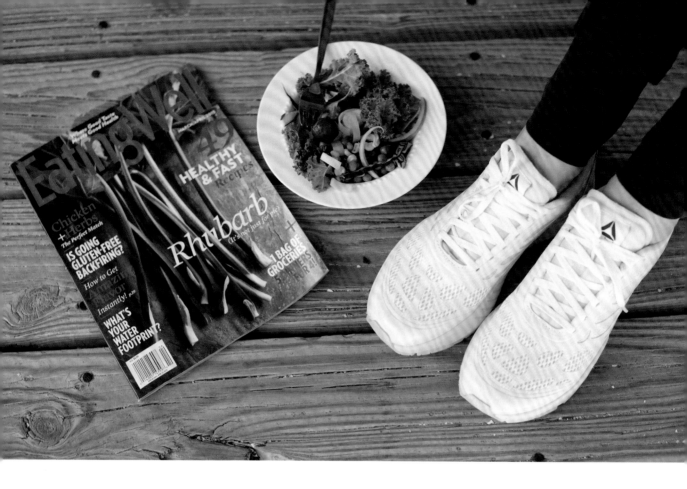

Week 3: Final week

To the right, you will find all you need for this week's recipes under the headings Dairy & Eggs, Dry Ingredients & Oils, and Vegetables.

For this week you will also need unrefined salt, black pepper, ground cinnamon, ground turmeric, vanilla powder, spirulina powder, dried oregano, dried thyme, vegetable stock cubes, tamari, baking powder, olive oil, coconut oil, tahini, ghee, coconut flour, almond flour, and Dijon mustard. These are basic ingredients so you may already have some of them in your kitchen. If something's missing, just add it to the shopping list.

Week 3: Shopping list

Dairy & Eggs
11 large eggs
1 cup (2½ dl) Greek yogurt
3½ oz (100 g) ricotta cheese
1½ cups (3½ dl) feta cheese
¾ cup (1½ dl) mozzarella cheese, grated
¾ cup fresh mozzarella cheese
1½ cups (3½ dl) Parmesan cheese, grated

Dry Ingredients & Oils
¼ tsp chili flakes
½ tsp poppy seeds
2 tsp hemp seeds
3 tbsp chia seeds
1 tsp sesame seeds
10 sweet almonds
1½ cups (3½ dl) almond milk
¼ cup (½ dl) tomato sauce, unsweetened
2 cups (4½ dl) coconut water
1 tbsp coconut flakes
1¼ cups (3 dl) chickpeas, cooked
10 olives
1 tbsp capers
1¾ cups (4 dl) quinoa
¾ cup (1 ½ dl) green lentils
4 sheets nori

Vegetables
2 lbs (950 g) spinach
1 yellow onion
4½ avocados
5 lemons
1 butternut squash
1½ garlic cloves
2 tomatoes
2 eggplants
7 carrots
3 celery stalks
3½ hothouse (English) cucumbers
1 corn on the cob, uncooked
1 yellow bell pepper
1¼ cups (3 dl) broccoli
1 generous lb (500 g) kale
2⅓ inch (6 cm) fresh ginger
1 large beet
1 cauliflower
3½ oz (100 g) mushrooms
fresh basil
fresh parsley
¼ cup fresh chives
¼ red onion
5 asparagus spears

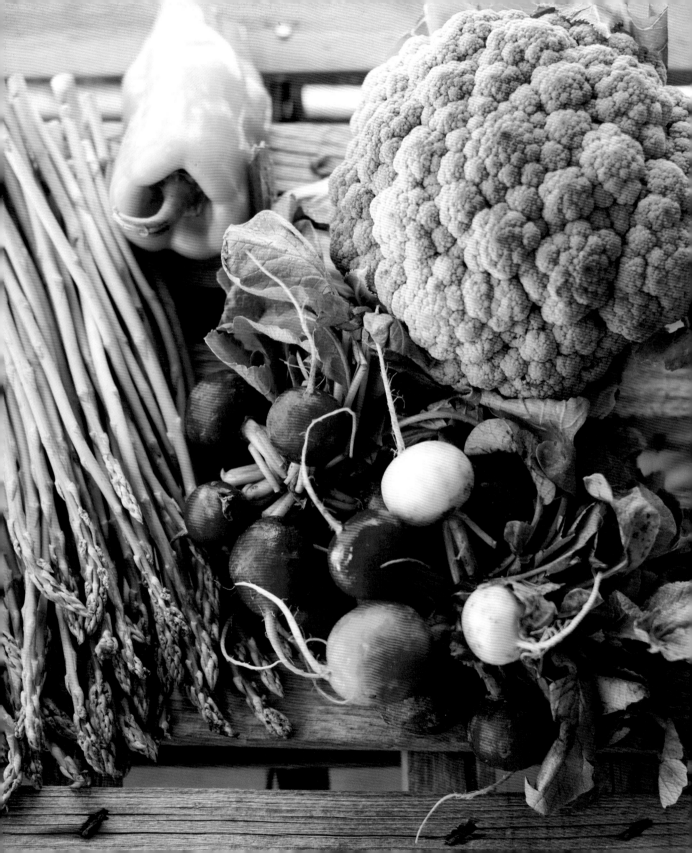

CHAPTER 5

Recipes

IN THIS SECTION YOU'LL FIND QUICK AND DELICIOUS VEGETARIAN DISHES. THEY'RE RICH IN PROTEIN, GOOD-QUALITY FATS, VITAMINS, AND MINERALS— EVERYTHING YOUR BODY NEEDS TO LET GO OF ITS SENSITIVITY TO SUGAR. HERE IS, AMONG OTHER THINGS, AN ASSORTMENT OF GREEN JUICES, AN ARO- MATIC POWER LOAF, WARM CAULIFLOWER PIZZA, AND CRISPY LETTUCE TACOS.

THE FOLLOWING PAGES ARE LOADED WITH FLAVORFUL VEGETARIAN RECIPES that were created exclusively for the sugar detox program. They're rich in protein, good fats, vitamins, and minerals—everything your body needs to let go of its sensitivity to sugar. The recipes are designed to help you on your journey and to make every turn on the road an easy one. You'll be reaching the finish line before you know it.

The dishes are vegetable-based, as they're the starting point of any clean and nutritious meal. Add a few extra vegetables or some fish if you feel your body needs something more, and don't forget to only use high-quality ingredients. You'll enjoy things like booster green juices and smoothies, coconut pancakes with ricotta topping, aromatic gluten-free bread, warm cauliflower pizza, and crispy lettuce tacos.

These recipes were inspired by different experiences in my life, as well as the various places where I grew up—Miami, New York, Westport, and New London. My mother has shown me the path to wholesome food, and has even contributed two recipes to this book—the butternut squash soup, and her delicious almond cake. I'm grateful that my eating habits are accepted at home. It's important to understand that food habits are intensely personal. No single way is right for everybody, but there is a right way for you. Try out different approaches to see what works best for just you. If you're not 100 percent certain yet, start with these recipes. Good luck—you'll do great!

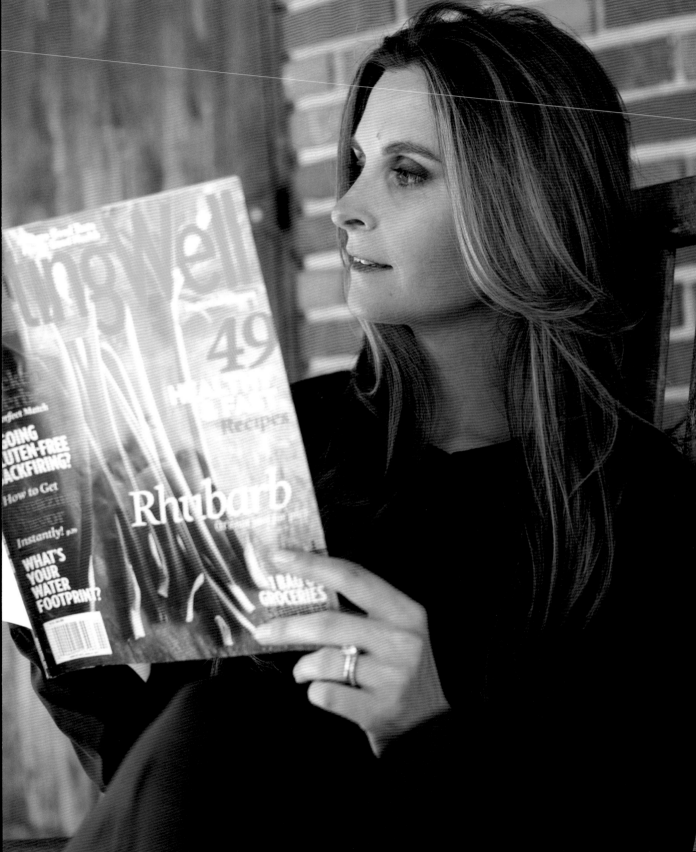

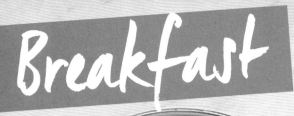

Breakfast

Lovely green smoothie

Protein muesli
with creamy yogurt

Coconut pancakes
with ricotta topping

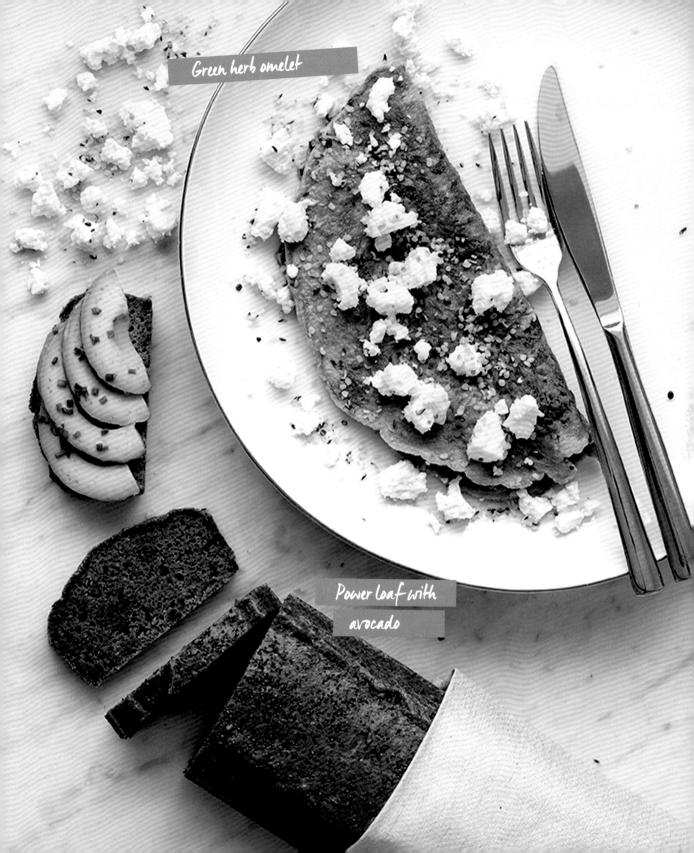

Green herb omelet

Power loaf with
avocado

Lovely green smoothie

SERVES: 1

Your body will love this wake-up call! Green is always a lovely color for breakfast. This smoothie contains protein, wholesome fats, vitamins, and minerals that you need to start the day off right.

½ avocado
1¼ cups (3 dl or 2 handfuls) spinach
½ cup (1 dl) broccoli
¾ cup (1½ dl) coconut water
¾ cup (2 dl) almond milk
1 tsp hemp seeds
freshly squeezed juice of ½ lemon

1. Mix all the ingredients to a smooth purée in a high-powered blender.
2. Pour into a glass and serve.

TIP!

If you prefer something warm in the morning, drink a glass of lukewarm lemon water 15 minutes before breakfast.

Coconut pancakes with ricotta topping

*Who doesn't love fluffy American pancakes for breakfast?
This recipe contains no sugar but is still full of flavor, so it's a good dish
to keep on hand after the end of the program; you can even add in some
coconut sugar if you feel okay doing so.*

¼ cup (½ dl) coconut flour
1 tsp baking powder
⅛ tsp unrefined salt
½ tsp vanilla powder
2 egg whites
½ cup (1 dl) almond milk
coconut oil, for frying
1 tbsp unsweetened coconut
  flakes
1 tbsp ricotta or Russian yogurt

1. Mix coconut flour, baking powder, salt, and vanilla powder in a bowl. Set aside.
2. With a fork, whisk the egg whites and the almond milk in a bowl. Add in the dry ingredients and mix thoroughly.
3. Heat 1 tsp coconut oil in a skillet, add the pancake batter, and fry the pancake on both sides. Add a few drops of oil to the pan for each pancake.
4. When serving, top the pancakes with coconut flakes and ricotta.

FACT
Coconut oil can help alleviate indigestion or a bloated stomach. It has antimicrobial properties and has a soothing effect on bacteria, candida, as well as parasites that have a detrimental effect on digestion. Coconut oil can also help calm irritable bowel syndrome (IBS).

Protein muesli with creamy yogurt

SERVES: APPROX. 10

This is the perfect quick grab-and-go breakfast! You can also have it for a snack at work. It's easy to pour the yogurt into a glass and sprinkle the crispy mix over the top. Once the program is over you can top it with some berries.

2 tbsp coconut oil
1 cup (2½ dl) unsweetened
  coconut flakes
¼ cups (½ dl) sesame seeds
1½ cups (3½ dl) sweet almonds
1½ cups (3½ dl) walnuts
1 tsp ground cinnamon
1 tsp ground cardamom
½ tsp unrefined salt

To serve
¾ cup (1½ dl) Greek or Russian
  yogurt, per serving
Optional: 1 tsp coarsely ground
  flaxseed, per serving

1. Preheat the oven to 255°F (125°C). Line a baking sheet with parchment paper.
2. In a bowl, mix all the dry ingredients with the coconut oil. Spread the mixture onto the prepared baking sheet. Place the sheet in the oven and bake for 20 minutes until the mixture is golden brown.
3. Let the muesli cool. Serve it with yogurt and top with coarsely ground flaxseed.

TIP!
This muesli will keep for about 2 weeks. Pour the week's servings into a container with a lid, and freeze the rest.

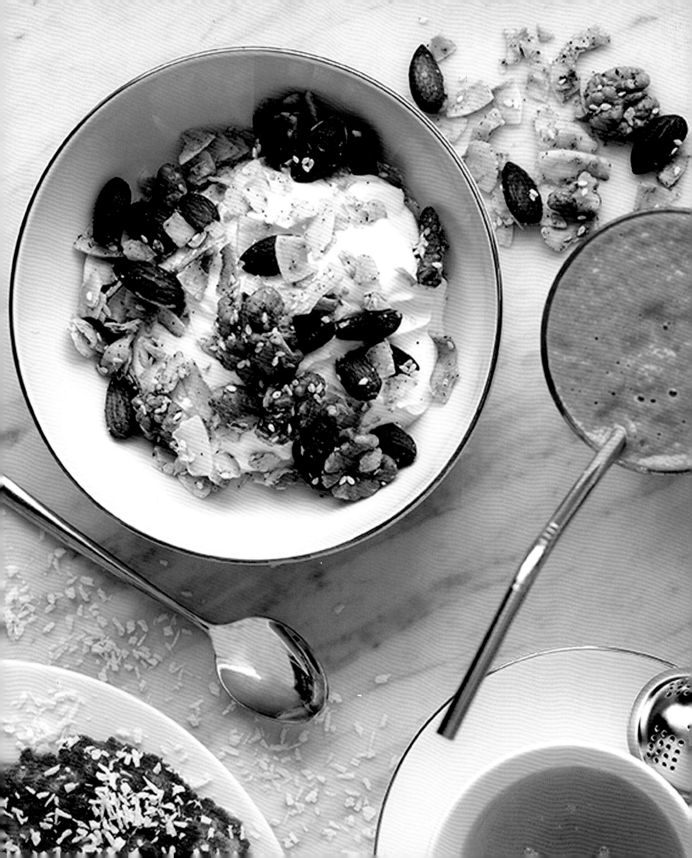

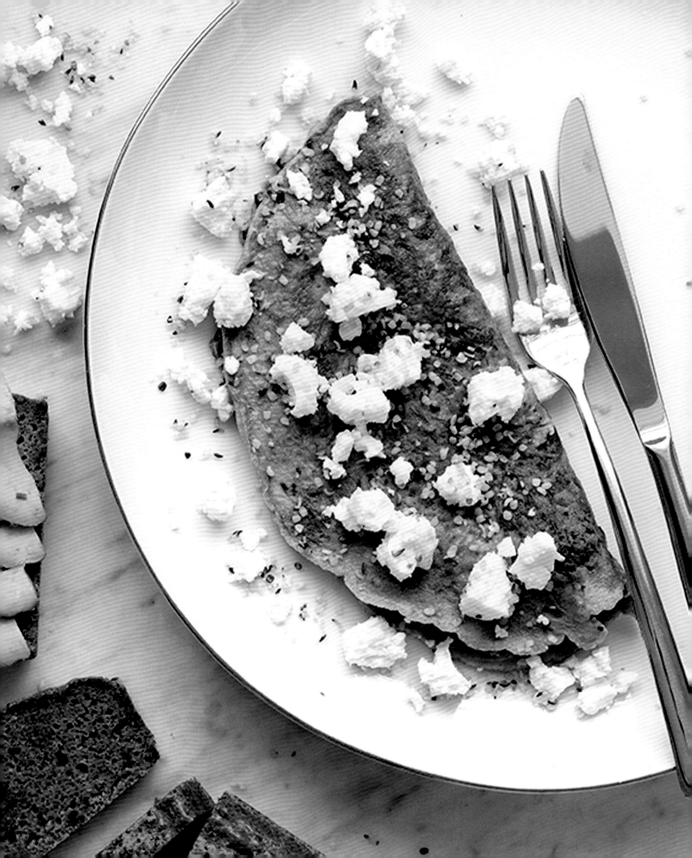

Green herb omelet

This breakfast imparts serenity and energy to your body for the day. You will feel just the right amount of full. The spirulina algae will give you a boost of vitamin B_{12}; you can mix in an extra ½ teaspoon of spirulina if you're used to it and enjoy the combination of flavors.

2 large eggs

1 tbsp water

¼ cup (½dl) fresh chives, finely chopped

½ cup (1 dl) broccoli, finely chopped

¼ tsp spirulina powder

1–2 handfuls of spinach, finely chopped

1 pinch unrefined salt

1 tsp coconut oil

2 tbsp feta cheese

1. Whisk together the eggs and water.
2. Mix the chives, broccoli, spirulina powder, and spinach in a bowl. Stir it into the eggs.
3. Cook the omelet in the coconut oil. Crumble feta cheese over the omelet when ready to serve. You can also add some extra spinach on the side.

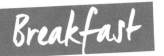

Power loaf with avocado

MAKES: 10-12 SLICES

You don't have to miss bread on this journey—it's included! This is a better option than store-bought loaves, because it's made with love as well as fewer processed ingredients. The bread goes well with a teaspoon of almond butter or sliced tomato, a drizzle of olive oil, and some freshly ground black pepper on top.

coconut oil, for the pan
1 cup (2½ dl) raw almond butter
4 large eggs, separated
¼ cup (½ dl) water
2½ tsp white wine vinegar
¼ cup (½ dl) buckwheat flour
1 tsp baking powder
½ tsp unrefined salt
1 tsp poppy seeds
½ avocado

To serve

1. Preheat the oven to 300°F (150°C). Prepare a loaf pan by oiling it with coconut oil.
2. Whisk together the almond butter and egg yolks, then add the water and the vinegar. Beat the egg whites in a separate bowl.
3. Mix buckwheat flour, baking powder, and salt. Add the dry mix to the almond butter/egg yolk mix and blend thoroughly. Fold in the egg whites. Pour the batter into the loaf pan and sprinkle poppy seeds on top. Set in the oven and bake for 35 minutes. Let the bread cool in the loaf pan before serving. Enjoy 2 slices for breakfast, either toasted or as is. Slice or mash the avocado, and put onto the sandwich.

Healthy scrambled eggs

Eggs contain many important minerals such as iron, zinc, and phosphorus. Research indicates that eating eggs can help protect against breast cancer, so eat your eggs with a clear conscience. Besides, they will keep you satiated for longer due to their good fats and protein.

2 large eggs
unrefined salt
black pepper
1 tsp coconut oil
¼ yellow onion
2 handfuls of spinach
3 tsp Parmesan cheese, grated
¼ tsp chili flakes

1. Mix the eggs with a pinch of salt and some pepper.
2. Melt the coconut oil in a skillet. Add onion and sauté until it has softened.
3. Add the eggs and spinach to the skillet, and stir for 1 minute.
4. Add the Parmesan cheese and chili flakes. Stir until the eggs are firm, and serve.

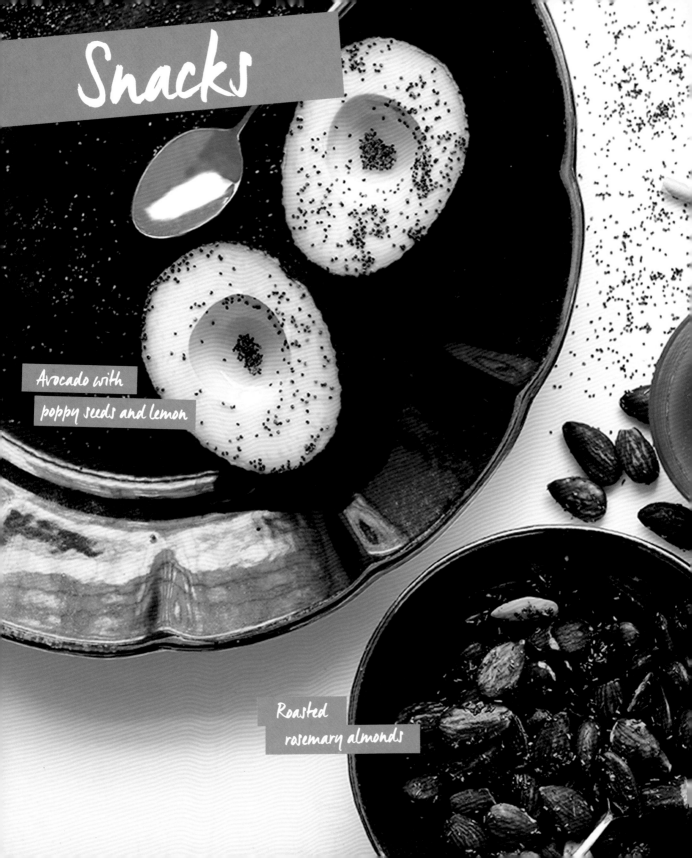

Snacks

Avocado with
poppy seeds and lemon

Roasted
rosemary almonds

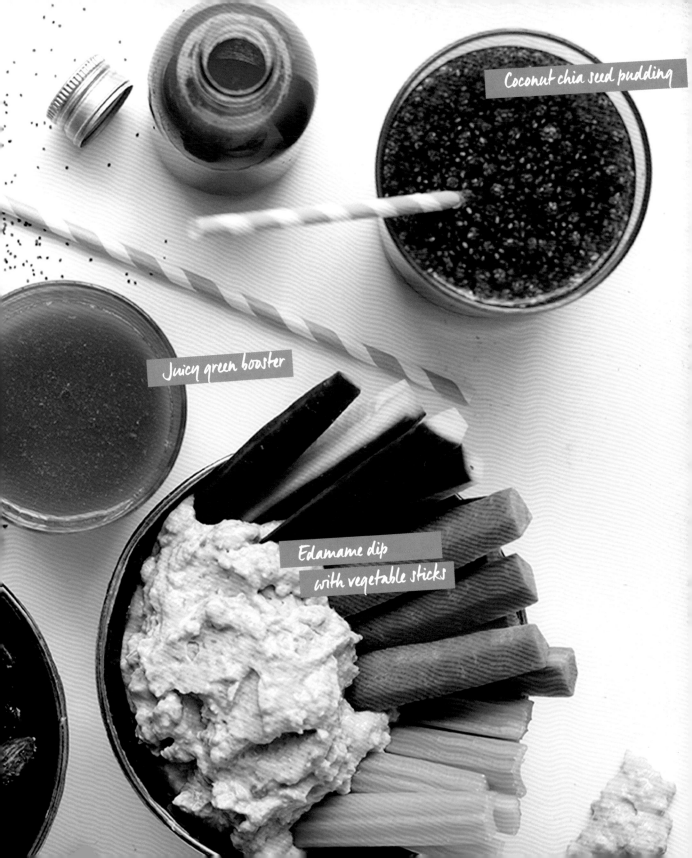

Coconut chia seed pudding

Juicy green booster

Edamame dip
with vegetable sticks

Coconut chia seed pudding

SERVES: 1

Chia seed pudding is a popular snack, as well as a health trend that seems to be here to stay. In this recipe the chia seeds are mixed with coconut water instead of milk, which means that this pudding contains all the protein, good fats, and extra electrolytes needed by anyone who enjoys an active lifestyle. You can even use this as an energy drink, before the texture changes and becomes thicker.

1 cup (2½ dl) coconut water
3 tbsp chia seeds
1 tsp vanilla powder
1 tsp ground cinnamon

1. Combine all ingredients together; let the mix sit in the refrigerator overnight, or until the texture has thickened and becomes jellylike.

TIP!

*Once you've finished the program you can add
a few berries to this pudding if you wish.
Raspberries make an especially nice addition.*

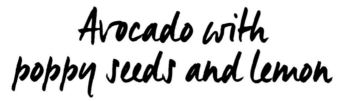

Avocado with poppy seeds and lemon

SERVES: 1

This simple snack is loaded with fiber—about $\frac{1}{3}$ oz (10 g) per serving—to fill you up and stabilize your energy in the afternoon. This creamy fruit (yes, this is a fruit you're actually allowed to eat while following the program) combines beautifully with some lemon juice and poppy seeds. It's a perfect snack to have at work—you can keep everything stashed in your desk drawer.

½ **avocado**
freshly squeezed juice of ¼ lemon
½ **tsp poppy seeds**
pinch of unrefined salt

Cut the avocado in half and remove the pit. Drizzle the lemon juice over the flesh, and sprinkle with some poppy seeds and salt. It's ready to eat!

FACT
Is the avocado not quite ready to eat yet? Put it in a paper bag for 2 to 4 days to hasten the ripening process. You can add a ripe banana to the bag to speed it up even more.

Edamame dip with vegetable sticks

SERVES: 2–3

You get to choose which vegetables you want to enjoy with this creamy green dip. Try carrots, celery, cucumber, or even broccoli. Why not offer this to friends and family on a cozy evening—it's a much healthier option than candy and chips.

12½ oz (350 g) edamame (soy beans), shelled
1 avocado, peeled and diced
¼ cup (½dl) water
½ cup (1 dl) Greek yogurt
wedge of lemon
½ garlic clove, peeled
1 tsp unrefined salt

To serve:
1 carrot
1 celery stalk
½ hothouse (English) cucumber
1 tsp olive oil

1. Pour the edamame and some salt into a saucepan of boiling water. Reduce the heat and let simmer 5 minutes.

2. Rinse the beans under cold water and mix in a food processor. Add avocado, water, yogurt, lemon, garlic, and salt. Pulse until you have a smooth purée.

3. Cut the vegetables into sticks. Pour the amount of dip you need for your snack. Drizzle olive oil over the dip and serve with the vegetables.

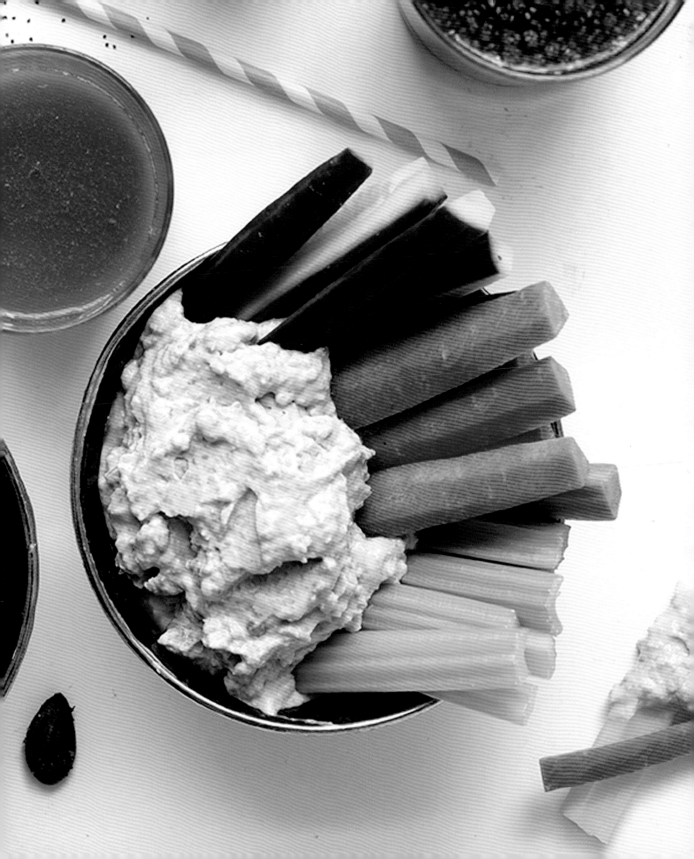

Juicy green booster

SERVES: 1

Consuming green juices and smoothies is one of the best things you can do for yourself. You'll quickly notice your body's positive response. When you drink greens your digestive system works better, your energy increases, and your skin becomes radiant. Your whole system gets the benefit of a chlorophyll-charged boost, along with a long line of vitamins and minerals. If you find it hard to swallow greens without any fruit, try adding some extra lemon and ginger to the recipe.

8¾ oz (250 g) spinach
8¾ oz (250 g) kale
1 carrot, peeled
1 celery stalk
1 hothouse (English) cucumber
1 lemon, peeled
1 1/5 inch (3 cm) fresh ginger

Cut up all vegetables. Blend in a high-powered blender. Serve in a pretty glass.

TIP!

If you still feel hungry after drinking the booster, eat a boiled egg. However, don't forget to figure out if this is real hunger before you decide to chow down on more food.

Roasted rosemary almonds

SERVES: ABOUT 10

Warning! You can become hooked on these savory, rosemary-infused roasted almonds. They are the perfect snack—you can carry them in a jar in your purse so you're ready when hunger strikes. The almonds provide the right type of energy by having both protein and good fat.

8¾ oz (250 g, 1¼ cups, 4 dl)
  sweet almonds
2 tsp coconut oil
1 tsp dried rosemary
1 tsp unrefined salt

1. Preheat the oven to 350°F (175°C). Line a baking sheet with parchment paper.
2. Mix almonds, coconut oil, and rosemary. Spread the mix on the prepared baking sheet.
3. Bake for 10 to 15 minutes, or until you start smelling a wonderful aroma from the oven. Remove the baking sheet from the oven and let the almonds cool for 20 minutes. Mix with salt and serve.

Lunch/Dinner

Butternut squash soup
with roasted squash seeds

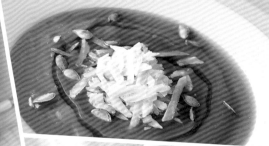

Colorful
quinoa bowl

Artichoke
with herb ghee

Brussels sprout salad with
Parmesan cheese and fried garlicky mushrooms

ENGLISH TEXT

DECOR
ITALIA

25 YEARS

LIGHT
LIVIN

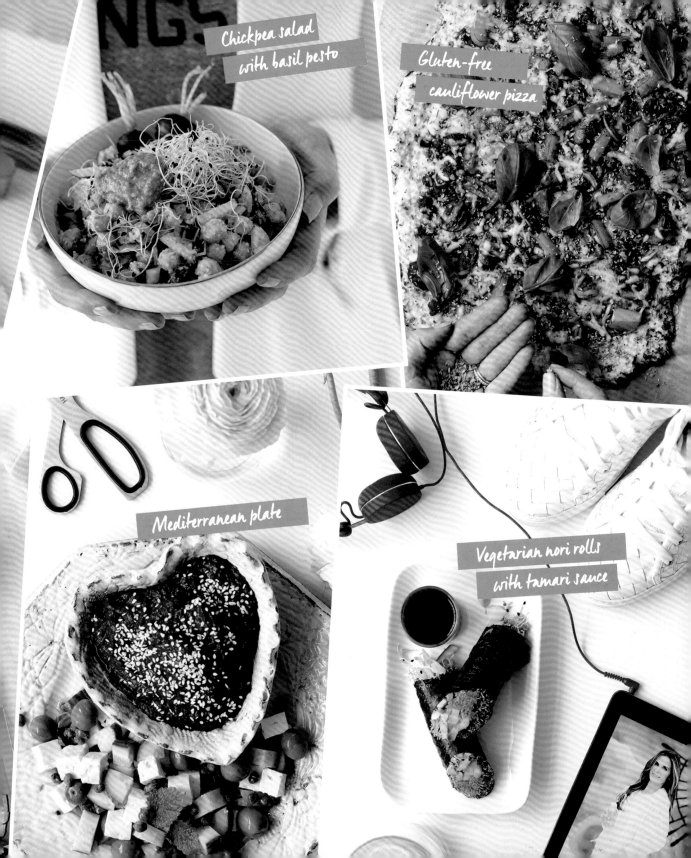

Chickpea salad
with basil pesto

Gluten-free
cauliflower pizza

Mediterranean plate

Vegetarian nori rolls
with tamari sauce

Colorful quinoa bowl

SERVES: 2

This is a simple and nourishing meal that can be prepared in 15 minutes. For a warm entrée try roasting the red onion and Brussels sprouts in the oven. You can also mix things up by using other vegetables, cheeses, nuts, and seeds. Use whatever you find in the refrigerator.

2 beets, peeled
2 carrots, peeled
1 avocado, peeled
½ small red onion, peeled
10 Brussels sprouts
3 tbsp feta cheese
2½ tbsp olive oil
freshly squeezed juice from
    ½ lemon
½ garlic clove, crushed
½ tsp unrefined salt
black pepper
1¾ cups (4 dl) quinoa, cooked
1½ tsp roasted poppy seeds

1. Grate the beets and carrots. Scoop out the avocado flesh, chop the onion, Brussels sprouts, and feta cheese.
2. Mix together olive oil, lemon juice, garlic, salt, and pepper as a dressing.
3. Place quinoa, vegetables, and feta cheese in a bowl and pour over the dressing and top with poppy seeds.

TIP!

If you want to eat this dish for lunch the next day, don't slice up the avocado, and leave the dressing off until it is time to eat.

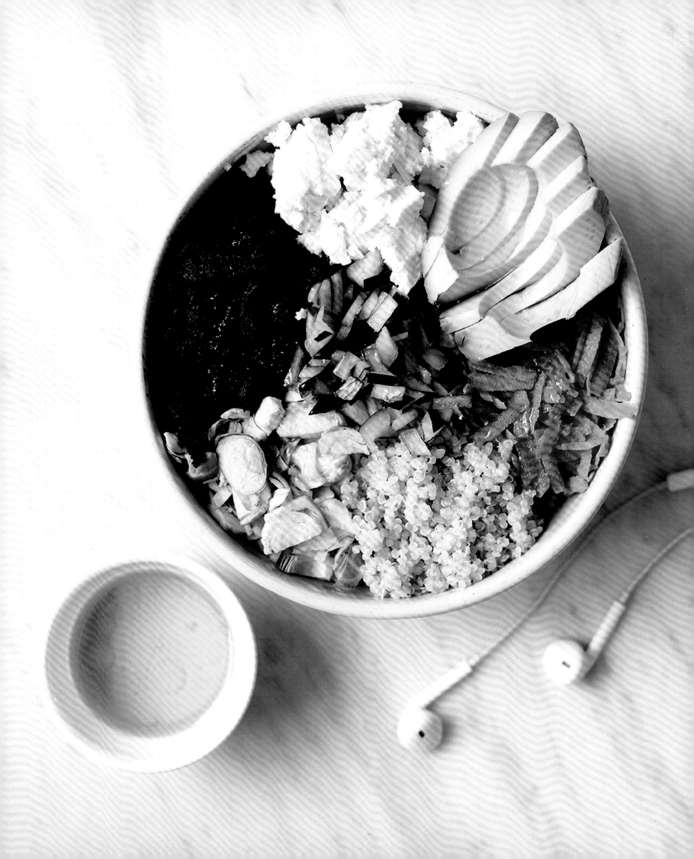

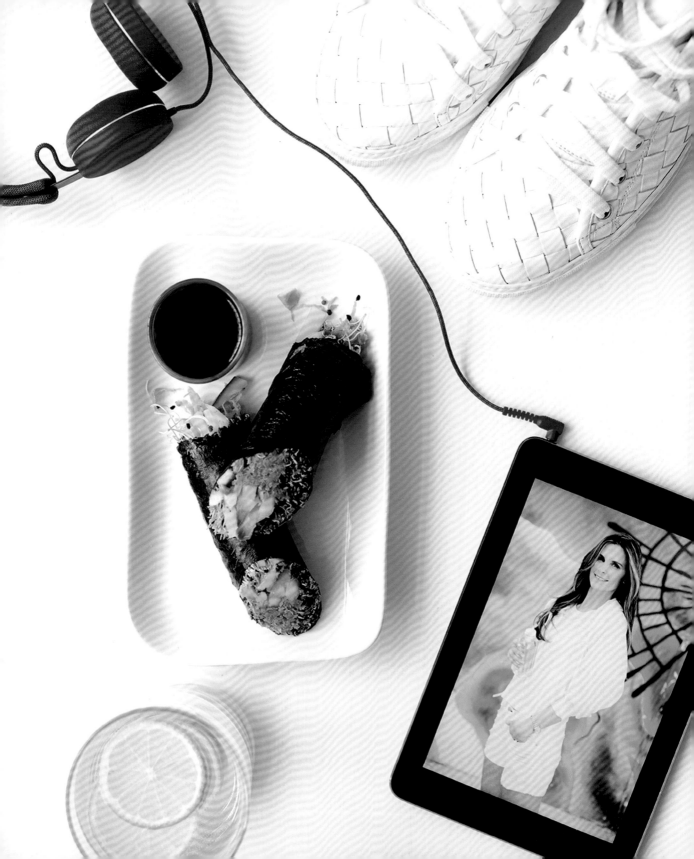

Vegetarian nori rolls with tamari sauce

SERVES: 2

Sea vegetables are incredibly nutritious, especially the awesome algae called nori. Did you know that as little as 3½ oz (100 g) nori contains 88 percent of your daily iron requirement? So now it's time to make your own vegetarian sushi; it's much easier than it looks.

2 carrots, peeled
½ hothouse (**English**) cucumber
1½ avocados
1¾ cups (4 dl) quinoa, cooked
4 sheets nori
½ lemon
3–4 tbsp tamari soy sauce

1. Grate the carrots and cut the cucumber into thin sticks. Slice the avocados into thin wedges.
2. Spread the quinoa, cucumber, carrots, and avocados over one side of the nori sheet. Start rolling up the sheet while rubbing the outer surface with the lemon. Continue rolling until the whole sheet is used.
3. Serve 2 rolls with tamari sauce. Prepare the rolls fresh for lunch, or the sheets will become tough.

TIP!
Try adding some salmon or other fish to the rolls.

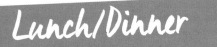

Root vegetable hash with spinach

SERVES: 2

An updated classic dish that is sure to please the whole family. Dice the vegetables and the haloumi cheese as small as you can. It's perfect for next day's brown bag lunch.

2 sweet potatoes, peeled
2 carrots, peeled
1 zucchini
7 oz (200 g) haloumi cheese
3 tsp olive oil
½ tsp unrefined salt
1 tsp dried rosemary
4 handfuls of spinach

1. Finely dice sweet potatoes, carrots, zucchini, and haloumi cheese.
2. Spread the olive oil onto a skillet; add in the diced vegetables and cheese. Sprinkle with salt and rosemary. Sauté until the chunks are soft and nicely colored. Serve with the spinach.

Flavorful corn frittata

SERVES: 2

Turmeric is hot these days, for a variety of reasons. Here it gives a frittata a bit extra "oomph."

½ yellow onion, peeled
1 tsp coconut oil
4 large eggs
¼ cup (½dl) almond milk
1 ear of corn, uncooked
½ yellow bell pepper
½ tsp ground turmeric
unrefined salt
black pepper
2¾ oz (75 g) ricotta

1. Preheat the oven to 350°F (175°C).
2. In a skillet, sauté the onion in some coconut oil until it is nicely browned. Whisk together the eggs and almond milk.
3. Cut off the corn kernels from the cob. Chop the bell pepper.
4. Mix the vegetables, turmeric, salt, and pepper with the egg/almond milk batter. Pour into a baking pan and dot the surface with ricotta. Bake in the oven for 15 to 20 minutes. Serve immediately.

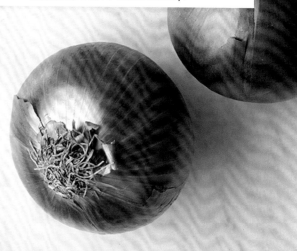

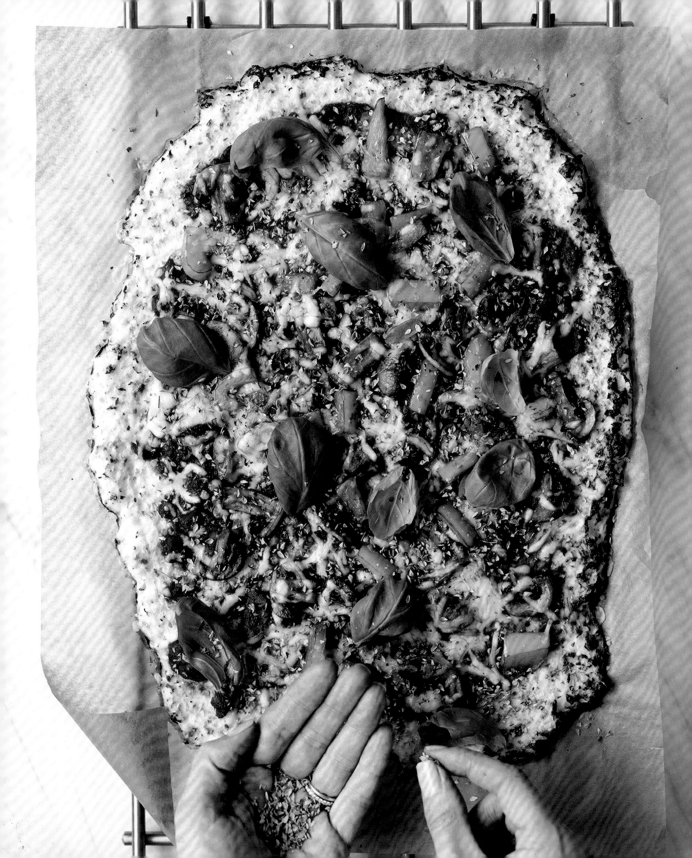

Gluten-free cauliflower pizza

SERVES: 2

Here at last is a gluten-free pizza, complete with characteristic Italian flavors of tomato, mozzarella, oregano, and basil. Avoid that heavy feeling, all too common after eating a traditional pizza, and enjoy feeling energized instead.

1 small cauliflower
2 large eggs
¾ cup (1½ dl) mozzarella cheese, grated
¾ cup (1½ dl) Parmesan cheese
½ tsp unrefined salt
3½ oz (100 g) mushrooms
½ yellow bell pepper
¼ cup (½dl) unsweetened tomato sauce
1 tsp dried thyme
1 tsp dried oregano
fresh basil, for topping

1. Preheat the oven to 430°F (220°C). Line a baking sheet with parchment paper.
2. Grate the cauliflower and mix it with eggs, ½ cup mozzarella, Parmesan, and salt.
3. Spread the dough into 2 round pizzas on the prepared baking sheet. Bake in the oven for 15 minutes.
4. While the pizzas are baking, sauté the mushrooms in a skillet, in coconut oil. Chop the bell pepper into small chunks.
5. When the pizza rounds are ready, spread some tomato sauce over them, and then layer on the fried mushrooms, bell pepper, thyme, oregano, ¼ cup grated mozzarella, and fresh basil. Return the pizzas to the oven, and bake for 3 more minutes, or until the cheese has melted.

Brussels sprout salad with Parmesan cheese and fried garlicky mushrooms

SERVES: 2

Most people choose to cook Brussels sprouts, but they are just as delectable when eaten raw, especially when combined with Parmesan and garlicky mushrooms. This fresh, flavorful dish is quick to make.

12½ oz (350 g) mushrooms
½ yellow onion
1½ garlic clove
coconut oil, for frying
30 Brussels sprouts
¼ cup (½dl) raw tahini paste
⅛ cup (¼dl) water
½ tsp freshly squeezed lemon juice
½ tsp unrefined salt
½ cup (1 dl) Parmesan cheese, grated
Your choice of sprouts

1. Clean off and chop the mushroom in chunks. Peel and finely chop the onion and the garlic clove.

2. In a large skillet, sauté the onion and garlic in coconut oil. Add the mushrooms and sauté for a few minutes until everything is soft and nicely browned.

3. Grate or julienne the Brussels sprouts into slim strips, and set them aside in a bowl.

4. In a blender, mix tahini paste, water, lemon juice, salt, and ½ garlic clove. Stir this dressing into the grated Brussels sprouts.

5. Add the Parmesan to the Brussels sprouts. Add the mushrooms on top and then the sprouts (this picture features beet sprouts).

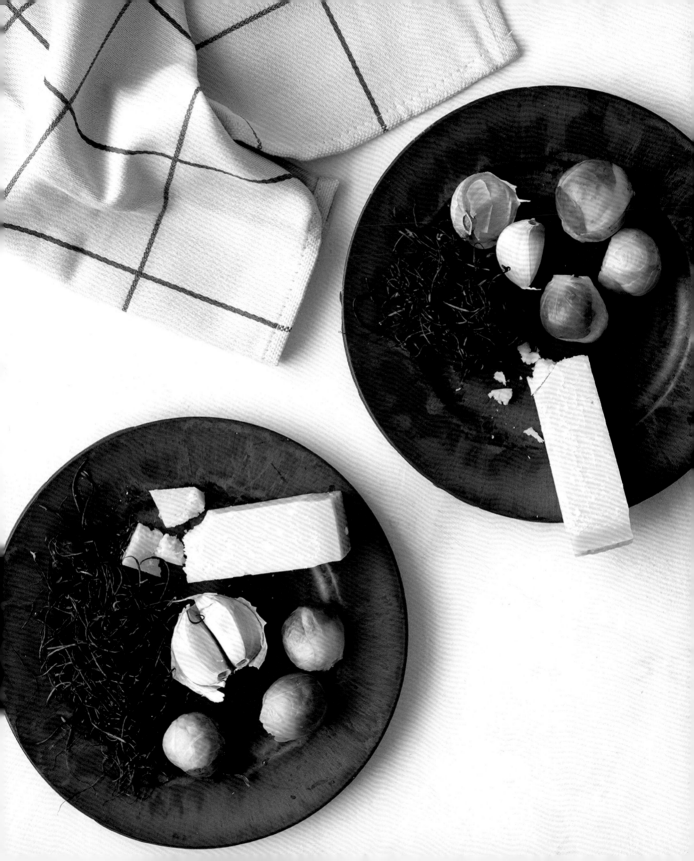

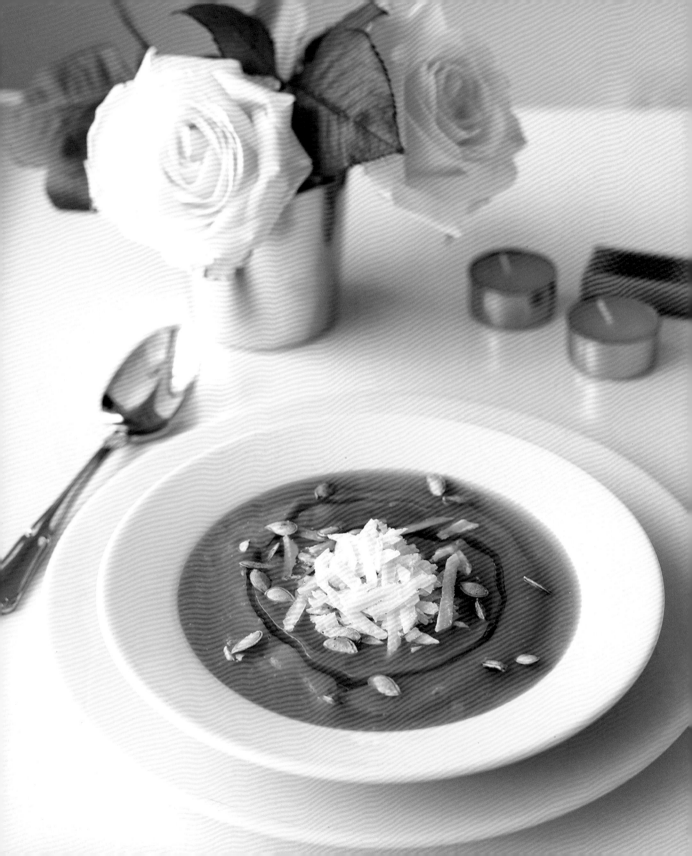

Butternut squash soup with roasted squash seeds

SERVES: 4

Soup is so simple to make, yet is such a nutritious meal. Best of all, you can make a double batch and freeze the leftovers for later. It's a perfect dish for those days when you're short on time but still yearn for a warm meal.

1 butternut squash
2 cups (5 dl water)
1 vegetable bouillon cube
unrefined salt
black pepper
2 tbsp squash seeds (use the
   ones from the butternut)
olive oil
4 tbsp Parmesan cheese, grated

1. Preheat the oven to 350°F (175°C).
2. Cut the squash in half across the middle and scoop out the seeds (save 2 tbsp seeds for the topping). Bake the squash for 30 minutes, or until the inside of the squash is soft.
3. In a large saucepan, bring the water to a boil along with the bouillon cube. Season with some salt and pepper. Scoop out the flesh from the squash and add it to the water; blend it with an immersion blender.
4. Roast the squash seeds in a skillet.
5. Pour the soup into a soup bowl. Add to it a few drops of olive oil, some grated Parmesan, and roasted squash seeds.

TIP!
To save time you can buy the seeds already roasted.

Quinoa fritters with green bean fries

SERVES: 2

This is a meal that completely satisfies all senses. I love making this dish on weekends when I have time to enjoy both the preparation of the dish and its flavors more fully.

8¾ oz (250 g) green beans
1 tbsp olive oil
unrefined salt
black pepper
1 small zucchini
1 small yellow onion, peeled
1 tbsp parsley
3½ tbsp coconut oil + extra
   for frying
1 cup (2½ dl) quinoa, cooked
3 large eggs
¼ cup (½ dl) almond meal
¼ cup (½ dl) yogurt, Russian
   or Greek
½ tsp freshly squeezed
   lemon juice

1. Preheat the oven to 435°F (225°C).
2. Trim the beans and place them in a baking dish. Drizzle some olive oil over them, and season with salt and pepper. Roast in the oven for 10 to 12 minutes.
3. Grate the zucchini. Finely chop the onion and parsley. Mix 3 tablespoons coconut oil, quinoa, eggs, almond meal, zucchini, onion, parsley, salt, and pepper.
4. In a skillet, melt 1 teaspoon of the coconut oil. Scoop up a large table-spoonful of the quinoa mixture and cook on both sides until golden brown. Continue with the remainder of the mix. You might need to add more coconut oil to the pan between fritters.
5. Mix yogurt, lemon juice, salt, and pepper to make a sauce. Add a few drops of olive oil on top. Stir until the sauce is smooth.
6. Serve 3 fritters with green beans and yogurt sauce per serving. You can freeze the leftover fritters for later.

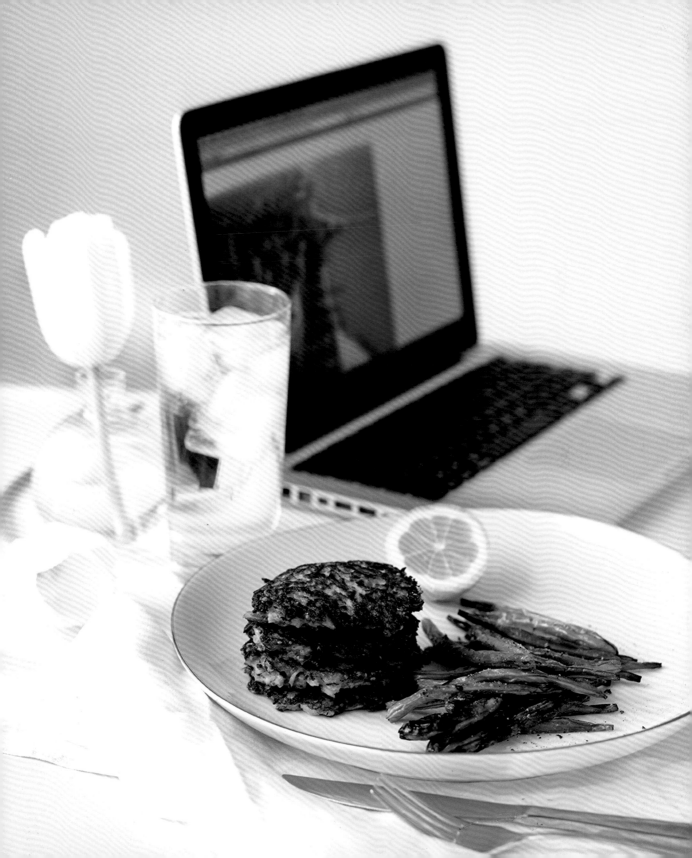

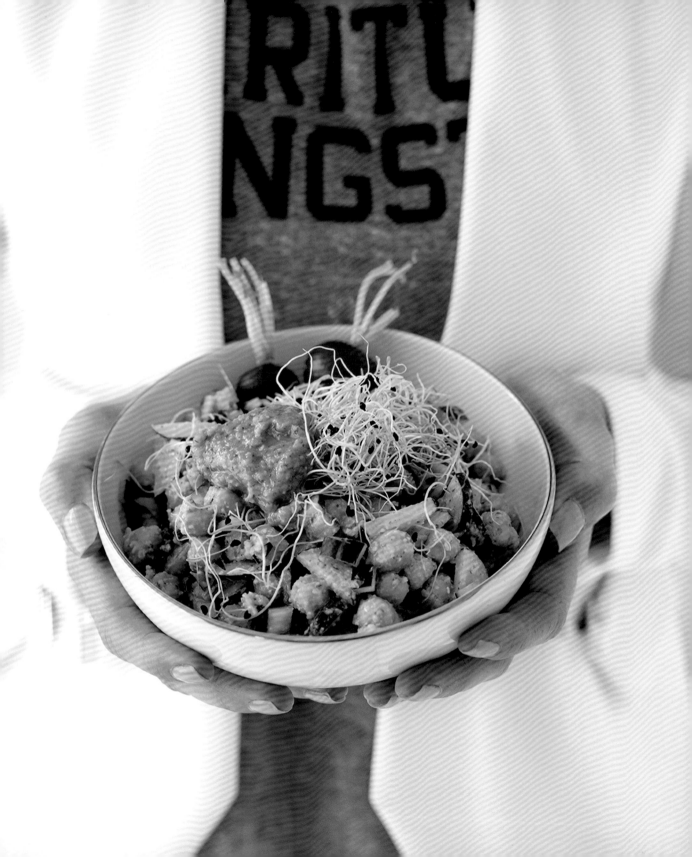

Chickpea salad with basil pesto

SERVES: 2

This is my version of a classic salad that was served at a lunch counter not far from my high school in Miami. I used to eat this salad several times a week. The chickpeas and homemade pesto make a perfect combination.

1¾ cups (4 dl) chickpeas, cooked
1 red bell pepper
8 radishes
¼ red onion
1 garlic clove
1 bunch of fresh basil
¼ cup (½dl) pine nuts
¾ cup (1½ dl) Parmesan cheese, finely grated
¼ cup (½dl) olive oil
unrefined salt
black pepper
Your choice of sprouts, for serving

1. Place chickpeas in a medium bowl. Chop the bell pepper, radishes, and red onion. Add to chickpeas.
2. Mash the garlic clove through a press. Mix the basil and garlic in a bowl. Add this to a food processor and mix with the pine nuts, grated Parmesan, and olive oil.
3. Pour the pesto over the chickpea salad, season with some salt and pepper, and toss everything together thoroughly. Serve with sprouts.

TIP!

Save any leftover pesto in the refrigerator. It will keep for up to 1 week.

Baked sweet potatoes with fresh ginger filling

SERVES: 2

Sweet potatoes contain magnesium, which is a calming, anti-stress mineral. This is my favorite recipe for fall. It'll give your immune system a real boost!

2 sweet potatoes
5¼ oz (150 g) white beans, cooked
¾ cup (2 dl) ricotta
⅓ inch (1 cm) fresh ginger, peeled and grated
1 tbsp freshly squeezed lime juice
lemongrass, chopped
1 tsp unrefined salt

1. Preheat the oven to 390°F (200°C). Line a rimmed baking sheet with parchment paper.
2. Prick the potatoes all over with a fork. Place them on the prepared baking sheet and bake them in the oven for 45 to 60 minutes, or until they are soft. Remove the potatoes from the oven and let them cool down a little.
3. Mix beans, ricotta, grated ginger, lime juice, lemongrass, and salt. Cut the potatoes in half down the middle, and spoon some of the ginger mixture on top. You can add more lime and ginger if you prefer a stronger flavor.

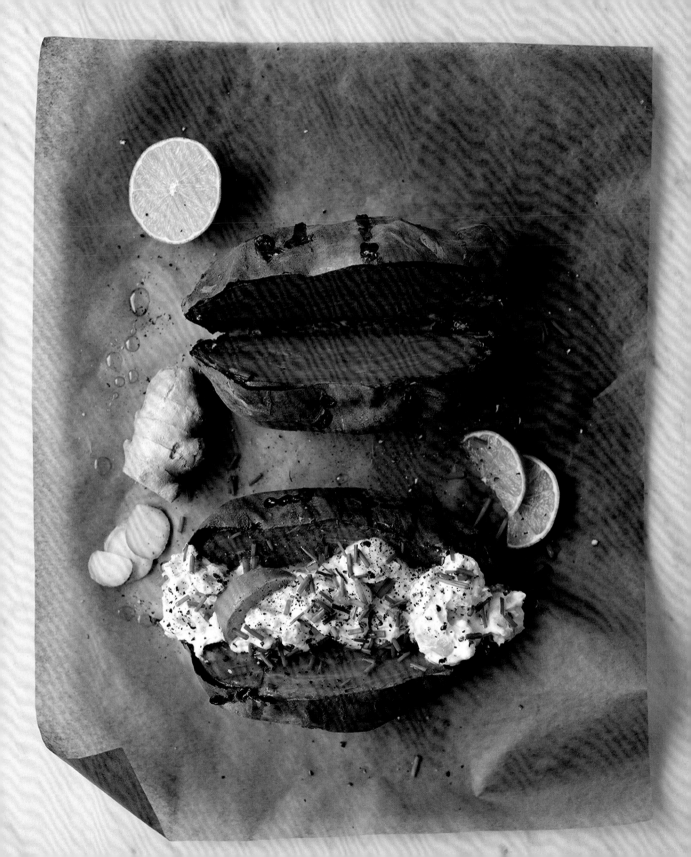

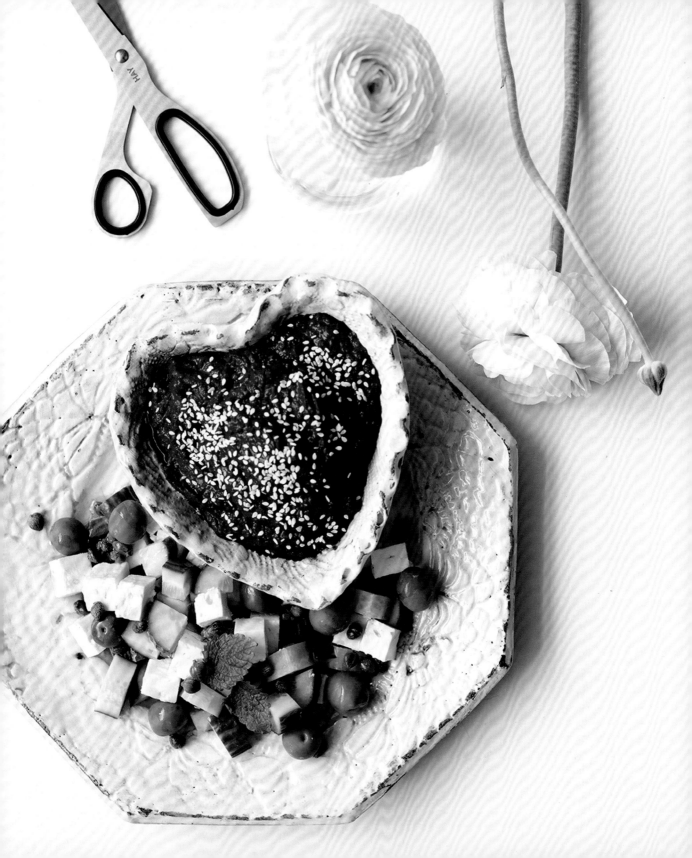

Mediterranean plate

SERVES: 2

There are some days when you just want to run down to the deli and pick up something tasty for dinner, like this Mediterranean-inspired combo. How about some creamy beet hummus, and light cucumber salad with feta, olives, and capers?

1 large beet
1¼ cup (3 dl) chickpeas, cooked
1½ tbsp olive oil
1 tbsp raw tahini paste
1 garlic clove, crushed
1 tbsp water
½ tsp unrefined salt
¼ tbsp lemon juice
1 tsp sesame seeds
½ hothouse (English) cucumber
6 tbsp feta cheese
1 tbsp capers
10 olives, pitted

1. Peel and cut the beet into smaller chunks. In food processor, mix it with chickpeas, olive oil, tahini, garlic, water, salt, and lemon juice. Transfer to a plate and sprinkle the hummus with sesame seeds.
2. Chop the cucumber and mix it with the feta, capers, and olives.
3. Serve on individual plates.

Spicy oven-roasted eggplant

SERVES: 2-3

Eggplant contains vitamins, minerals, and fiber, which makes it a great addition to salads, stews, and oven-baked dishes like this one. Spice up your life with some chili, and enjoy the heat of the spice when combined with fresh tomatoes and mozzarella.

2 eggplants
2 tomatoes
³/₄ balls of mozzarella cheese
3 tbsp olive oil
½–1 tsp unrefined salt
½ tsp chili powder

1. Preheat the oven to 400°F (200°C).
2. Cut the eggplants in half lengthwise and place them in an oven dish, cut-side up.
3. Drizzle with olive oil; season with salt and chili powder on the cut side. Bake in the oven for 30 minutes, or until the eggplants are soft.
4. Slice tomatoes and mozzarella, and spread over the eggplant. Return dish to the oven and bake for another 5 minutes.

Lettuce tacos with chili-flavored cauliflower rice & creamy guacamole

SERVES: 2

My husband loves tacos, so we try to come up with recipes that work for carnivores and vegetarians alike. He usually makes the classic version, while I choose to skip the corn taco shell and fill a large, lovely lettuce leaf with healthy ingredients instead. Food is a personal journey, but that shouldn't prevent you from eating together.

¼ head cauliflower

¼ tsp chili powder

2 avocados

unrefined salt

½ tsp freshly squeezed lemon juice

1½ tomatoes

¼ hothouse (English) cucumber

¼ red onion

4 large lettuce leaves (romaine, for example)

1. Finely grate the cauliflower. Mix with the chili powder.
2. Scoop out the avocado flesh and mash it with a fork. Mix the mash with some salt and squeezed lemon juice to make a creamy guacamole. Finely chop tomatoes, cucumber, and red onion.
3. Fill lettuce leaves, and enjoy.

Artichoke with herb ghee

SERVES: 2

This simple dish is both fresh and filling. It's best to cook the artichoke the day you're going to eat it, and I recommend that you eat them slowly and savor each leaf. This is a good example of mindful eating.

2 artichokes
2 tbsp ghee
1 pinch of unrefined salt
black pepper
½ garlic clove, crushed
chives, chopped
power loaf (see page 86)

1. Rinse the artichokes and cut off their stems. Bring salted water to a boil in a saucepan and place the artichokes in the water. Cook them for 30 to 40 minutes, depending on their size.
2. Mix the ghee, salt, pepper, garlic, and chives.
3. Drain off the water from the artichokes. Transfer them to a platter together with the herb ghee. Enjoy with 1 or 2 slices of power loaf.

FACT

Ghee is clarified butter, and is beneficial for eyesight, skin tone, memory function, and digestive health. It can be found at well-stocked grocery stores and online.

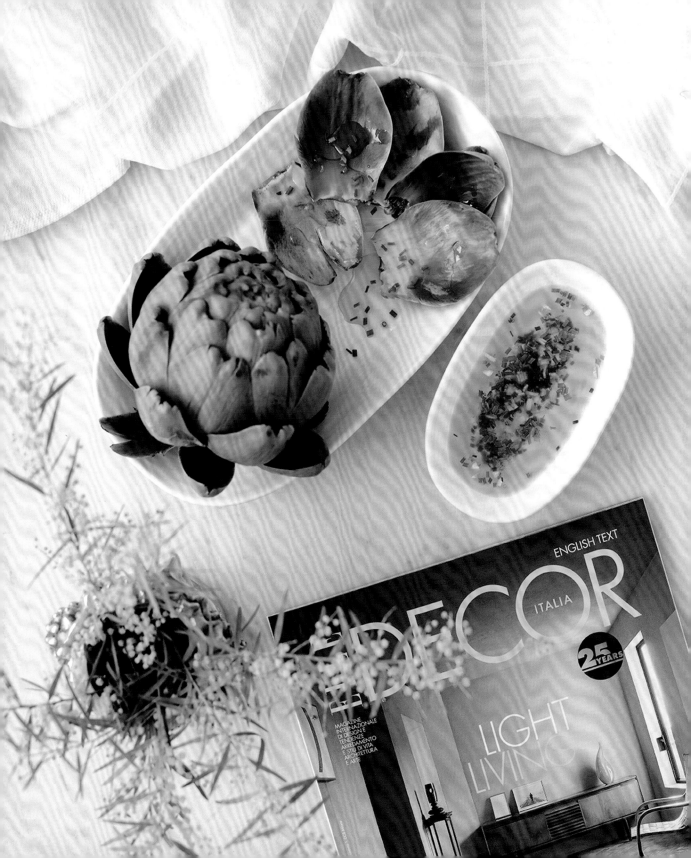

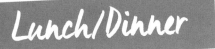

Red hot Thai curry

SERVES: 2

You can substitute other vegetables in this recipe. Add in what you already have at home, or try the combination below. Give your body a health boost with plant-based food!

1 tbsp coconut oil
1 garlic clove, peeled and chopped
1 yellow onion, peeled and chopped
⅓ inch (1 cm) fresh ginger, peeled and chopped
1 head broccoli, chopped
1 zucchini, chopped
1 red bell pepper, chopped
1 carrot, peeled and chopped
½ cup (1 dl) green peas
3½ oz (100 g) mushrooms, chopped
14¼ oz (400 ml) can coconut milk
1½ tsp red curry paste
1½ tsp ground turmeric
1 tsp ground cinnamon
freshly squeezed juice from ½ lime

1. Melt the coconut oil in a saucepan and sauté garlic, yellow onion, and grated ginger.
2. Add in all the vegetables, mushrooms, coconut milk, curry paste, spices, and lime juice.
3. Bring to a boil, lower the heat, and let simmer for 15 to 20 minutes. Serve.

Warm lentil salad with oven-roasted vegetables and feta

I love hearty salads that keep me full for a long time. This recipe is for just such a salad. If you're really hungry, add in a piece of salmon.

2 carrots
½ red onion
10 asparagus spears
5–6 tbsp olive oil
1 pinch black pepper
1 tsp unrefined salt
1¼ cups (3 dl) green lentils
20 sweet almonds
¼ cup (½dl) parsley
¾ cup (2 dl) feta cheese
1½ tbsp Dijon mustard
2 tsp freshly squeezed lemon
  juice

1. Preheat the oven to 435°F (225°C).
2. Chop carrots, onion, and asparagus into small chunks, and transfer them to a roasting pan; drizzle them with 1 to 2 tablespoons olive oil. Season with salt and black pepper. Place in the oven and roast for 20 minutes.
3. Rinse the lentils and boil them in water for about 15 minutes. Set aside. Chop the almonds, parsley, and feta.
4. For the dressing, mix 4 tablespoons olive oil, Dijon mustard, lemon juice, and a pinch of salt.
5. Mix together the oven-roasted vegetables, lentils, and dressing. Top with almonds, parsley, and feta.

FACT

Lentils are a good source of iron, needed to transport oxygen efficiently through the body and increase energy. Other iron-rich foods include spinach, seeds, beans, nuts, Brussels sprouts, and eggs.

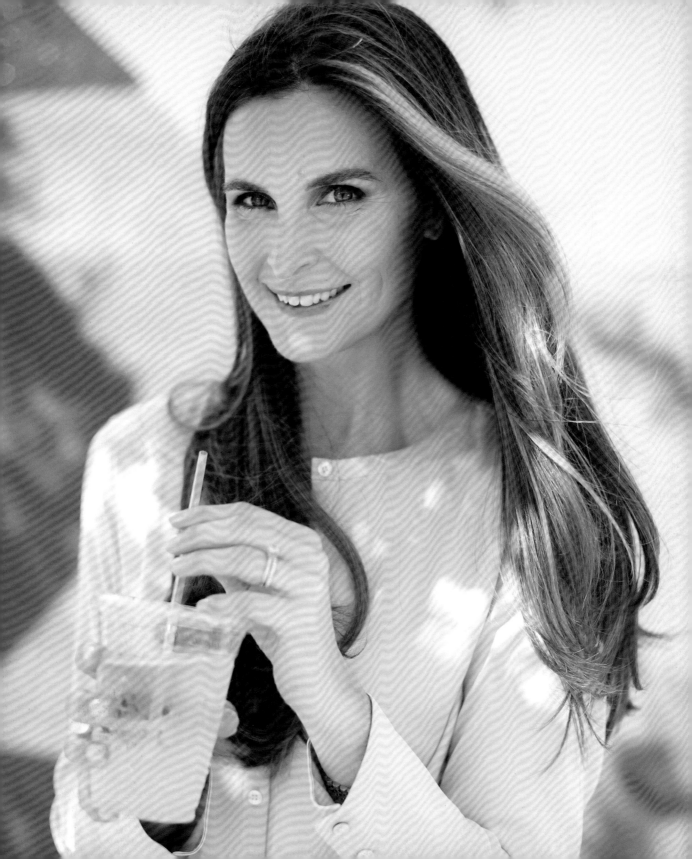

CHAPTER 6

Living a Healthy Lifestyle after the Program

CONGRATULATIONS—YOU'VE MADE IT! HOPEFULLY YOU'RE ALSO FEELING IN BETTER HEALTH. BUT WE'RE NOT DONE YET. THIS CHAPTER COVERS THE BEST CHOICES IN SWEETENERS; OFFERS ADVICE ON HOW TO GET BACK ON TRACK IF YOU ARE MOMENTARILY DERAILED; AND SHARES TIPS ON HOW TO KEEP HEALTHY HABITS FOR LIFE.

CONGRATULATIONS ARE IN ORDER—YOU HAVE COMPLETED THE PROGRAM AND SHOULD FEEL PROUD TO HAVE MADE IT TO THE END! How does it feel to be free from sugar, and to live without constant cravings for sweets? Surely this has been well worth the effort. By now you will have noticed all the wonderful benefits that come from laying off sugar for a while. Do you sleep better at night? Maybe you're experiencing an indescribable inner calm, while at the same time feeling a surge of energy? Does your skin look clearer? Are you more even-tempered? Are you finally able to avoid, or politely decline, the offer of sweets without feeling anxious? Even if you didn't make it through the full program, be proud of yourself. Just fire up the program once you feel up to it again—don't give up.

We all experience a range of benefits while undergoing a sugar detox. Some are more obvious than others. Do you remember the quiz "Are you sensitive to sugar?" on page 18? Return to it now and ask yourself those same questions; hopefully your answers will be completely different. Even if you only answer one less yes, be proud of yourself—it's not easy to let go of sugar. The cravings can be strong, but there's a huge sense of freedom when you can steer your thoughts away from sugar. I know how difficult it is to ignore those unsolicited negative thoughts that pop up—and they will continue to do this from time to time. After completing the program, your task is to let these thoughts float past like clouds—don't pay them any attention and don't let them take over again. Immediately say a positive affirmation or thought. Choose love over fear. There's no reason you shouldn't continue living this new lifestyle without sugar. You can do it!

Go back over the list of twenty-seven reasons not to eat sugar (on page 20). Your body is constantly working to create balance and optimal health, so do your best to help it along. Remember that sugar can cause inflammation, cellulite, dental cavities, depression, migraines, acne, sleep disturbances, decreased sex drive, fatigue, irritation, and cardiovascular disease—everything you should try to avoid. Say thanks, but no thanks to all that. Concentrate instead on what you want, and what you have probably already achieved while following the program. It's not worth the risk of developing any of the above

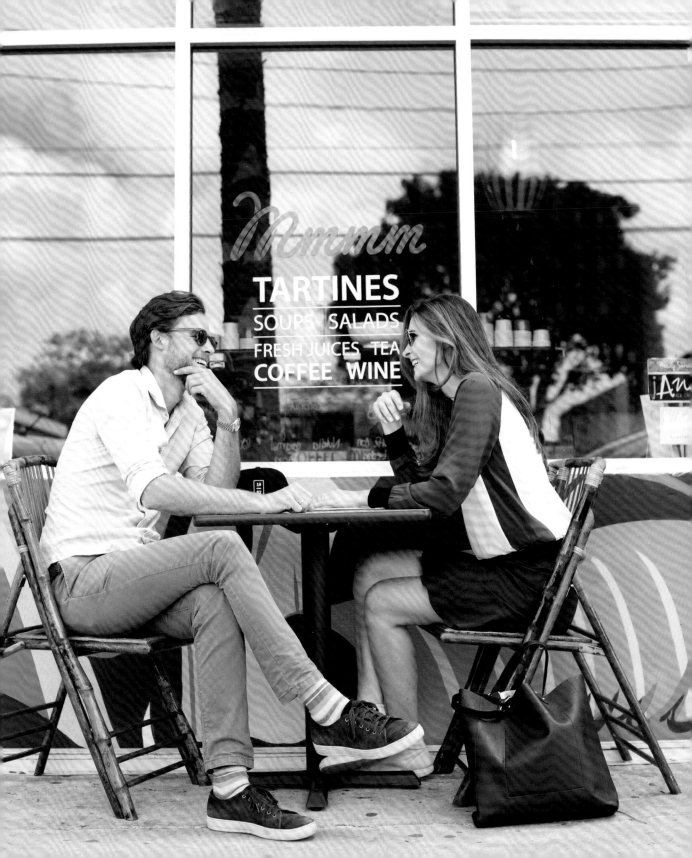

ailments for a fleeting taste of sweets on the tongue. It's worth decreasing your sugar intake so you can experience increased self-confidence; to have more even-keeled energy; to build a stronger immune system, and to increase your chance of fertility. You have managed to detox from a substance that has far-reaching negative effects on your life.

You can choose to continue living a sugar-free lifestyle a little while longer—it's entirely up to you. You're the master of your body, and hopefully these past three weeks will have taught you to read your body's signals more accurately and eat according to what your body needs. After all, only you know how your body prefers to be fueled. Only you have the answers. New research is constantly being published—and will be throughout our lifetime—advising us how to eat. All you can do is try these ideas out for yourself; if you feel confused, go back to the basic principles, and listen to your stomach and your intuition.

FIRST WEEK AFTER PROGRAM'S COMPLETION

You can try to carefully reintroduce some sugar to your meals in the first week after the program's completion, beginning with natural sugar in berries and fruit. Start with one serving of fruit per day, adding another serving if it feels right for you. Berries are ideal—blackberries, blueberries, raspberries, and strawberries are full of antioxidants, vitamins, and fiber. A big bonus!

Throughout this week continue to eat according to the rules of clean eating. Concentrate on unprocessed and organic produce that your body recognizes as food. Your body is now used to living without all the added sugar, and is sure to appreciate the boost in nutrition. You can combine this book's recipes with other similar ones, or with your own healthy favorites. You can also keep eating the meals from the program if that feels less risky to you, rotating the three weeks' worth of menus. If you'd like, you can add in some more food from meat and fish categories.

If you'd rather go back to your former routines and eating habits, I still recommend that you consume lots of vegetables, drink lots of water, and take it easy when reintroducing sweets to your meals. Eat what feels right for you, but remember to listen and feel your hunger; don't just head down to the nearest pizza joint for a large, toppings-heavy pie. You will be able to enjoy pizza from time to time, but try not to overload your system right off the bat with large portions. I want you to be able to enjoy the fruits of your labor, and the effort you put into following the sugar detox program. Plan your usual meals but in reasonable amounts, and deal honestly with your hunger pangs. What would you really like to eat? Ask yourself this question before every meal. Furthermore, avoid buying too many food products that have added sugar in them. It will be difficult to resist temptation if you go back to filling your pantry with candy and cookies. Start by buying healthier options such as fruit, sweets made from natural ingredients, and dark chocolate. Consider your choices carefully so you don't fill your shopping cart with sweet treats out of sheer habit. I can't recommend that you consume a lot of simple (white) carbohydrates either, since they turn to sugar very quickly once ingested. You can't go full-out on meatballs and mashed potatoes or spaghetti carbonara just because the program is over. Try some of the things you've missed the most, and see how you cope. Listen to your body and see how it reacts—it's as simple as that. Again, keep in mind that it's all about eating in moderation and paying attention to your body.

Start a new relationship with food

Continue to use your positive affirmations as a pep talk and guide. Perhaps you're ready for a new positive affirmation, now that the program is over. Write down your goals related to food, and choose whichever one is most significant to you. From this, you can create a fresh and motivating motto or affirmation for the rest of your nutrition journey in the months ahead. The psychological aspect of it is important and can help you stay on course. Remember: the words, thoughts, and energy you're emitting will come back to you one way or another, so use them to your advantage.

Remember: the eating habits you're creating are meant to last a lifetime. Don't settle on a diet that's too restrictive, and don't beat yourself up—keep up the loving relationship and respect for your health, even if you fall off the wagon at times. Slipping is entirely normal; there will always be dinner parties, birthdays, holidays, and other events where you won't be able to eat what is healthiest from your standpoint—and you know what? That's absolutely okay. When sugar has ceased to be a controlling factor, it's easier to savor a piece of cake and not become overwhelmed by cravings for sweets the next day. Maybe you can already handle eating chocolate, and feel entirely satisfied with only one small piece.

Give your natural detox system a helping hand!

Your internal detox system will still be active after the end of this program; there is no off switch there. What you have done over the past three weeks is help your body maximize its daily cleansing. We typically consume large amounts of unhealthy food, a load that our body then has to deal with. It rarely puts up a fight, all while doing its best to clean up the mess of sugar, heavy metals, bad bacteria, etc. When we make healthier choices we also help our system along in its cleansing work, the way it was built to function. We let our body perform a more thorough and deep cleansing, which reduces the inflammations that could cause serious illness.

Our lungs also play an important role in the detox process, as they help to eliminate toxins. We have to show our organs respect, and we can do this by eating nutrient-rich meals and making good choices in our daily diet.

Over the course of the program, the liver is not overtaxed, so keep helping it in its work of processing and cleansing. In tandem with the kidneys, the liver's job is to purify the blood, so for optimal liver function, eat clean and drink eight glasses of water (about 6½ cups or 1½ liters) per day. You'll ingest some fluids naturally through the food you eat. But if you don't often feel thirsty, or if you have a tendency to forget to drink, set a pitcher of water on your desk or on the kitchen table at home. If you're usually on the go, buy yourself a nice, leakproof water bottle that you can stash in your bag. Plain water can get boring after a while, but there are many flavors you can add to make it taste more exciting.

Try adding some of my favorite flavorings to your water:

- Mint leaves
- Raspberries and cucumber slices
- Lemon wedges and ice cubes
- Lime wedges and fresh strawberries
- Ice cubes made with watermelon juice
- Apple wedges and ground cinnamon
- Orange wedges and vanilla powder

SECOND WEEK AFTER PROGRAM'S COMPLETION

Once two weeks have gone by, you can try reintroducing honey, coconut sugar, chunks of dried fruit, and green stevia to your meals. Give my healthy desserts (found on pages 132–139) a try.

Good and bad sugar choices

Stay vigilant when you enter sugar's domain again, because bad choices lurk among the treats out there. They may leave a pleasant aftertaste on the tongue, but they can also have lingering, harmful effects on your body. You're probably more aware and cautious of hidden sugars after following this program, and you'll have more tricks up your sleeve when confronted with food choices in the future. Here are a few options you can turn to—all of them in moderation, of course. When or if you choose to eat something sweet, make sure to savor each bite. No bad conscience allowed!

Good choices
1. Dates
2. Fruit
3. Organic green stevia
4. Honey
5. Coconut sugar

Bad choices
6. Agave syrup
7. Aspartame (often found in light products and chewing gum)
8. Ethanol (in alcoholic beverages)
9. High fructose corn syrup (HFCS)
10. Sugar alcohols like xylitol, glycerol, sorbitol, maltitol, mannitol, and erythritol
11. White refined sugar

Healthy sweets

There are better alternatives when you feel you're ready to try something sweet!

Bake, mix, and create healthier sweets by using dates, coconut sugar, and honey as sweeteners. You'll find recipes for four of my favorite treats on the following pages.

Mom's almond and chocolate cake with poppy seeds

SERVES: 12

It was in her kitchen that my mom, Birgitta, came up with the recipe for this delicious almond cake. You never know how she's going to decorate it—it looks different every time she makes it. Put some time and effort into making a beautiful mosaic of nuts and dried fruit. Your guests are sure to beg you for the recipe.

1¼ cups (3 dl) sweet almonds
15 Medjool dates, pitted
½ tsp vanilla powder
1 pinch unrefined salt
1¾ oz (50 g) dark chocolate (85% cacao)
½ cup (1 dl) walnuts
¼ cup (½dl) dried apricots
1 tbsp poppy seeds
1 tbsp unsweetened coconut flakes

1. In a food processor mix ¾ cup (2 dl) almonds and all the dates. Add vanilla powder and salt. Spread the mixture onto a large plate; with your fingers, shape the mixture into a round, flat cake.

2. Melt the chocolate and spread it over the cake. Let the chocolate drip over the edge of the cake. Decorate the cake with nuts, dried fruit, poppy seeds, and coconut flakes while the chocolate is still soft.

3. Place the cake in the refrigerator to set for about 30 minutes before serving.

TIP!

This ingredients list is only a suggestion—you can use any combination of nuts or seeds that you prefer. The cake in the picture features pecans, pistachios, poppy seeds, almonds, and dates.

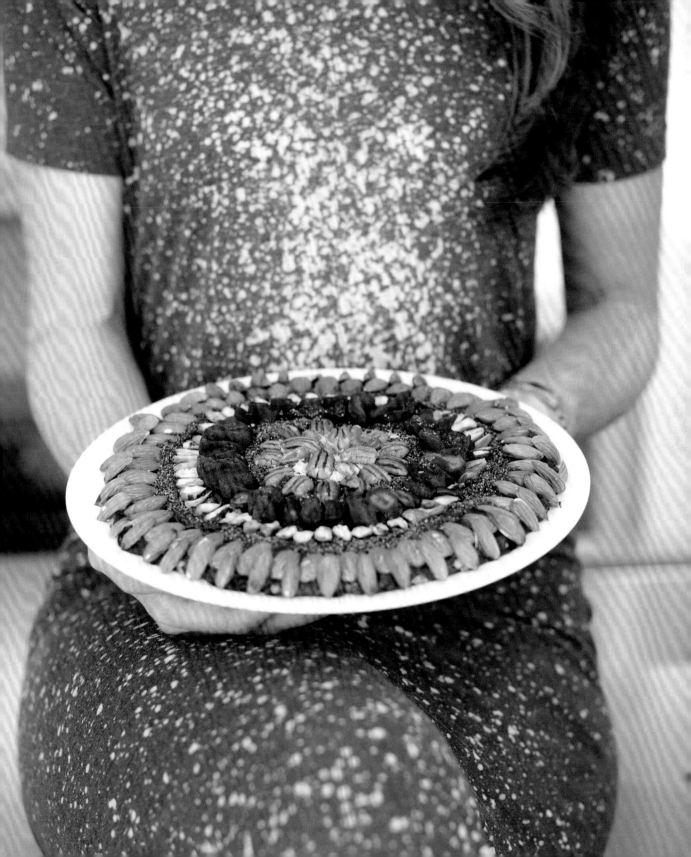

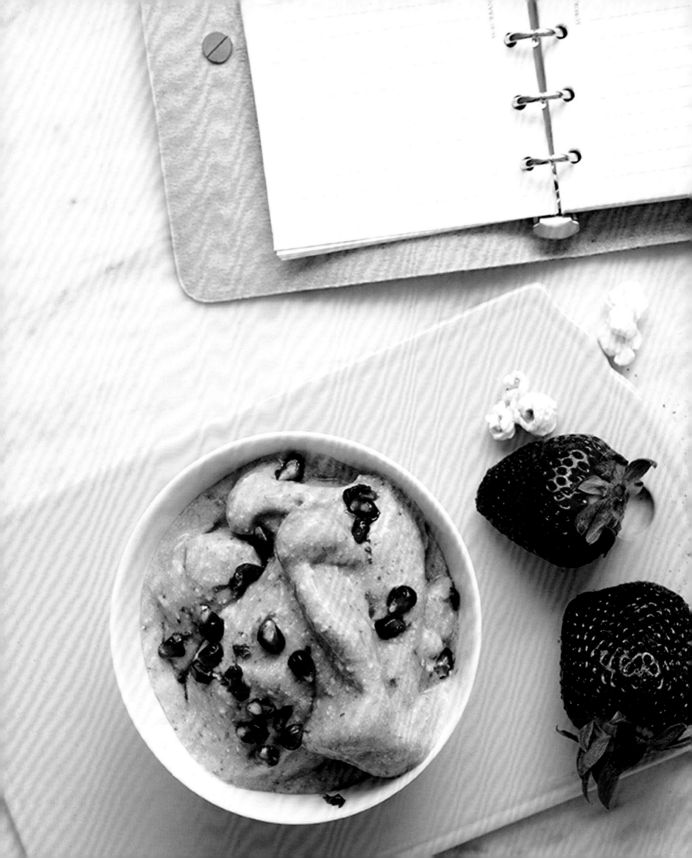

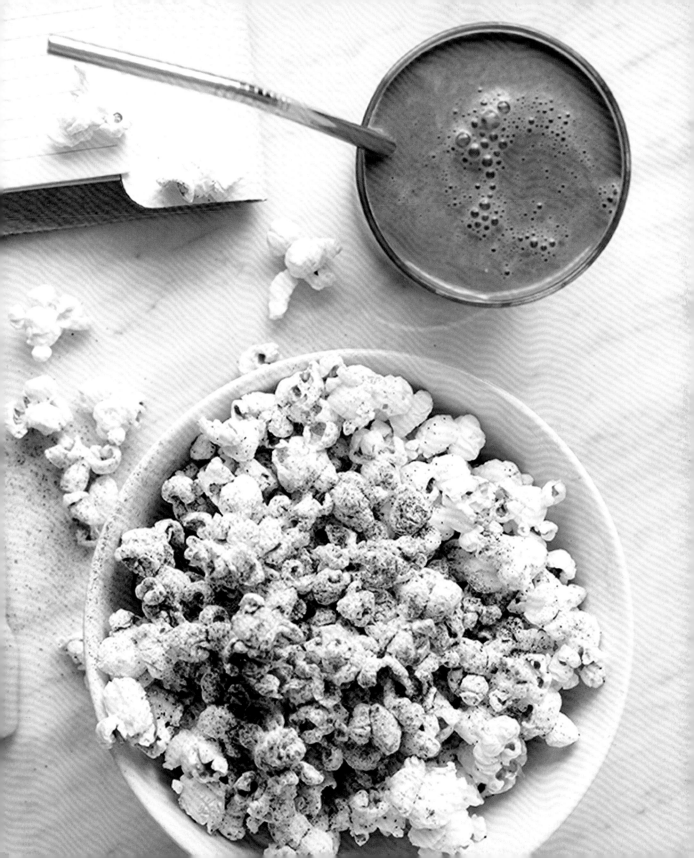

"Raw clarity" chocolate smoothie

SERVES: 1

This smoothie is a bestseller at my juice shop in Stockholm. It's creamy and full of flavor—a 100 percent pleasure for your taste buds. You're even getting some good-for-you fats and protein as an added bonus.

¾ cup (2 dl) cashew milk
2 tsp raw cocoa
2 Medjool dates, pitted
1 banana, frozen

Mix all the ingredients in a blender. Pour into a glass and serve.

FACT
Raw cocoa is a rich source of antioxidants, which fight free radicals that can cause harmful damage to the body.

Sweet cinnamon-flavored popcorn

SERVES: 2

Skip the microwaveable popcorn, which could be bad news for your health. Pop your own corn instead using coconut oil or ghee. Settle onto the sofa and enjoy some sweet popcorn with coconut sugar and salt. You can also make a bowlful without any toppings, or play around with other options you have on hand in your kitchen.

1 tbsp coconut oil
⅛ cup (¼ dl)
**   popcorn kernels**
½ tsp ground cinnamon
¼ tsp unrefined salt
1 tsp coconut sugar

1. In a saucepan, heat the oil over high heat. When the oil has melted, add in the corn kernels. Place a lid to the pan and listen to the kernels pop. Shake the pan occasionally to avoid burning the popcorn.

2. When all the kernels have popped, pour them into a bowl. Mix the cinnamon, salt, and coconut sugar together, and sprinkle over the popcorn.

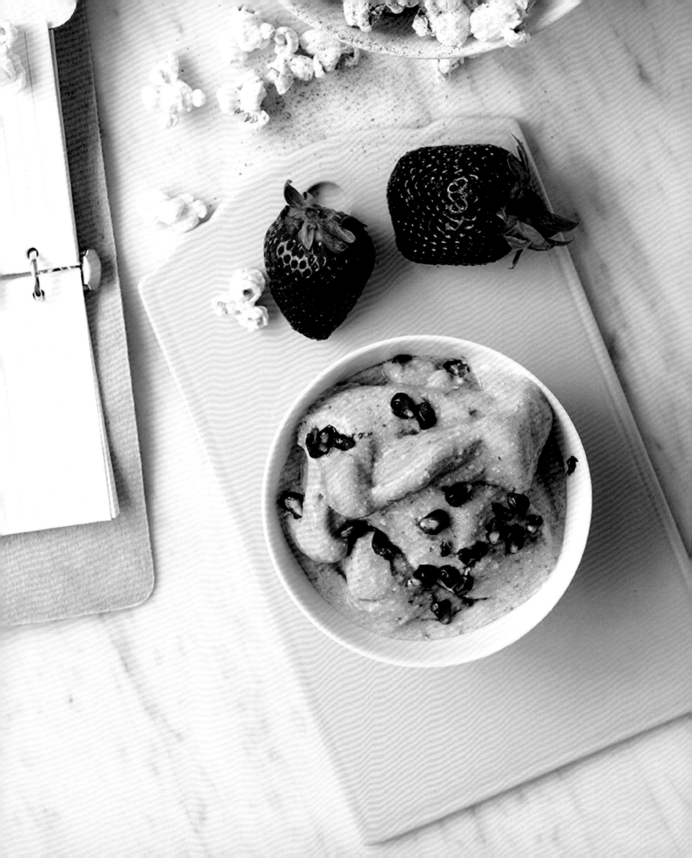

Strawberry ice cream

You scream, I scream, we all scream for ice cream! And yes, you can eat this with a clear conscience. Try this recipe with other berries if you like, such as raspberries and blueberries, or a mix of both—it's your call. This is a dessert you can enjoy year-round, not just in summer.

¾ cup (2 dl) coconut cream
¾ cup (2 dl) frozen strawberries
1 banana, frozen, peeled, and
  sliced
1 tbsp coconut sugar
½ pomegranate, seeds only

1. Pour the coconut cream, strawberries, banana, and coconut sugar into a blender. Blend to a smooth purée.
2. Scoop the ice cream into a bowl, and top it with pomegranate seeds.

HEALTHY HABITS FOR LIFE

Once again, congratulations on breaking free from sugar's stranglehold, and for choosing ingredients and meals that are healthy for your entire body instead. You can feel proud that you ignored all the sweets around you. It takes a psychologically strong person, and one who respects and cares for their body, to go twenty-one days without sugar. By now you will have a better understanding of what sugar is, and how it can damage your body and your health, so you'll have some thoughts on what your future relationship with sugar will be.

Relapse tips

So what happens if you relapse and your sensitivity to sugar returns? Don't worry, the following advice can help you get back on track again; you can always go back to the program, or make use of your favorite recipes to get your inspiration back.

1. Always plan your meals to leave no room for sweets.
2. Don't give up completely if you relapse at one particular point in time. Get back on track immediately! Let the next meal be healthy and clean.
3. Fill yourself up with vegetables, juices, soups, and smoothies.
4. Talk to someone who understands your situation. Chatting with a friend might just be enough to stave off a problem.
5. Try to find comparable options for the types of food you're craving. For example, if you yearn for a cinnamon bun, try some apple wedges smeared with peanut butter and sprinkled with cinnamon instead.
6. Remind yourself of your goals and what is genuinely important to you.
7. Say your positive affirmation aloud if a sugar craving hits, and remind yourself of how you really wish to feel and what to experience. Return to mindful eating, and be present while eating.
8. Write down ten reasons for not eating sugar.
9. Drink plenty of water—at least 6½ cups a day.
10. Don't skip meals, and eat at about 3 hour intervals to keep your blood sugar levels stable.

11. Make protein and good fats a part of each meal. This will also benefit your blood sugar levels, and make you feel satiated.
12. Make friends with Mr. Sandman, and get enough sleep every night.
13. Clean your kitchen of all sweet temptations. It's so much easier to stay on track when you don't keep treats at home.
14. Exercise. It will provide you with energy and focus.

Inspiration

Establish new habits for life to avoid sugar slumps, yo-yo dieting, and the latest diet craze, and concentrate instead on living your life to the fullest. Your body is perfect as it is. It is wise. It doesn't make mistakes. You don't have to tell it each day how much it should weigh. You don't need to overanalyze your food choices. You only have to notice how you react to what you eat and what signals your body is sending you. Listen to your inner you; you'll find all the answers there—yes, even regarding what to have for lunch today. Stay aware and don't disconnect from your gut feelings. It is your guide. Continue down that same road with the help of your trusty human GPS.

Say good-bye to sugar, and hello to health!

SOURCES

Appleton, Nancy and Jacobs, G.N. *Suicide by Sugar* (2009).

Quinn, Samantha. *The Real Truth About Sugar: Dr. Robert Lustig's "Sugar: The Bitter Truth"* (2012).

http://ngm.nationalgeographic.com/2013/08/sugar-cohen-text

http://www.netdoktor.se/traning-kost/nyheter/Svenskar-far-i-sig-40-kilo-socker-per-ar/

http://articles.mercola.com/sites/articles/archive/2012/02/22/how-sugar-accelerates-aging.aspx

http://authoritynutrition.com/10-disturbing-reasons-why-sugar-is-bad/

http://www.finely.fi

http://nancyappleton.com

http://drbenkim.com/articles-bloodsugar.html

http://www.theguardian.com/lifeandstyle/2014/aug/24/robert-lustig-sugar-poison

http://articles.mercola.com/sites/articles/archive/2014/12/10/sugar-porcessed-foods.aspx

http://www.huffingtonpost.com/kristin-kirkpatrick-ms-rd-ld/dangers-of-sugar_b_3658061.html

http://www.icakuriren.se/Test-Rad/Konsument/Lask-varsta-sockerfallan/

CONVERSION CHARTS

METRIC AND IMPERIAL CONVERSIONS

(These conversions are rounded for convenience)

Ingredient	Cups/Tablespoons/Teaspoons	Ounces	Grams/Milliliters
Butter	1 cup = 16 tablespoons = 2 sticks	8 ounces	230 grams
Cheese, shredded	1 cup	4 ounces	110 grams
Cream cheese	1 tablespoon	0.5 ounce	14.5 grams
Cornstarch	1 tablespoon	0.3 ounce	8 grams
Flour, all-purpose	1 cup/1 tablespoon	4.5 ounces/0.3 ounce	125 grams/8 grams
Flour, whole wheat	1 cup	4 ounces	120 grams
Fruit, dried	1 cup	4 ounces	120 grams
Fruits or veggies, chopped	1 cup	5 to 7 ounces	145 to 200 grams
Fruits or veggies, puréed	1 cup	8.5 ounces	245 grams
Honey, maple syrup, or corn syrup	1 tablespoon	.75 ounce	20 grams
Liquids: cream, milk, water, or juice	1 cup	8 fluid ounces	240 milliliters
Oats	1 cup	5.5 ounces	150 grams
Salt	1 teaspoon	0.2 ounce	6 grams
Spices: cinnamon, cloves, ginger, or nutmeg (ground)	1 teaspoon	0.2 ounce	5 milliliters
Sugar, brown, firmly packed	1 cup	7 ounces	200 grams
Sugar, white	1 cup/1 tablespoon	7 ounces/0.5 ounce	200 grams/12.5 grams
Vanilla extract	1 teaspoon	0.2 ounce	4 grams

Fahrenheit	Celsius	Gas Mark
225°	110°	$1/4$
250°	120°	$1/2$
275°	140°	1
300°	150°	2
325°	160°	3
350°	180°	4
375°	190°	5
400°	200°	6
425°	220°	7
450°	230°	8

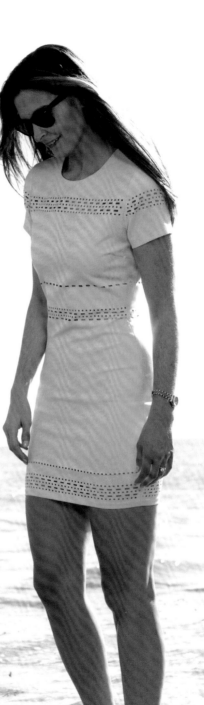

THANK YOU!

My Mom and Dad

My siblings, Gustaf, Ludde, Louise, and Eric

Marisol Flor Angela Duque Ariar

Gianina Ferrando

Anna Sjödin

Julia Fors

Monique Miller

Erika Billysdotter

Olle Svensson

Cecilia Viklund

Linnéa von Zweigbergk

Sanna Sporrong

Marie Jungsand

Karla Garcia

Ulrika Pousette

Alexis Garcia

Luca Mencarini

Intermix

Patriksson Communications

Monika Khavar from IbeyoStudio

AWB

JugoFresh

Mmmm Wynwood

Wynwood Shipping